May 7
Jackie's bday

Hoping for More

Hoping for More

Having Cancer, Talking Faith, and Accepting Grace

Deanna A. Thompson

FOREWORD BY
Krista Tippett

 CASCADE *Books* · Eugene, Oregon

HOPING FOR MORE
Having Cancer, Talking Faith, and Accepting Grace

Cascade Books
An Imprint of Wipf and Stock Publishers
199 W. 8th Ave., Suite 3
Eugene, OR 97401

www.wipfandstock.com

ISBN 13: 978-1-61097-981-8

Cataloging-in-Publication data:

Thompson, Deanna A., 1966–

Hoping for more : on having cancer, talking faith, and accepting grace / Deanna A. Thompson; foreword by Krista Tippett.

xviii + 148 p. ; 21.5 cm.

978-1-61097-981-8

1. Cancer—Religious aspects—Christianity. 2. Cancer—Patients—Religious life. 3. Cancer patients—United States—Biography. I. Tippett, Krista. II. Title.

BV4910.33 T46 2012

Manufactured in the U.S.A.

Author photo by Jennifer Skaptason

Contents

Foreword

WE TEND TO USE words like "miracle" and "mystery" in the context of serendipity. In this frank and eloquent account of life transformed by cancer, Deanna Thompson explores these articles of faith as they are also wont to appear, on the hard edges of hope and the dark side of joy.

I have known Deanna Thompson since we were both studying at Yale Divinity School in the early 1990s. She was a few years younger and headed for a career in academia. I was struck by the purity of her intelligence and joy. Then, we met again in Minnesota, where we both landed. I remember musing to myself at the good fortune of her students at Hamline University, where she became a professor. "Getting paid to talk about God is a pretty sweet deal," she writes, as this book opens. Her delight in the work of theology and the art of teaching was always evident and infectious.

The new conversation with God that she began after her diagnosis of Stage IV cancer is a conversation that countless people are having in our time. Medicine is sometimes in the business of documentable miracles, and maybe it will cure cancer one day. But for now, cancer in all its variety is a rampant reminder to modernity that we are mortal. Still, when it strikes a person as young and beautiful as Deanna Thompson, as full of promise, as beloved and necessary to her husband, young daughters, friends, and students, none of us can help but ask why.

This book is, in the first instance, one woman's memoir of the odyssey that a diagnosis of cancer becomes—a journey through a terrifying terrain of tests, hospital beds, medications, and treatments—of radical changes inside her body and in the ecosystem of her life.

Deanna Thompson's particular story is also, to be sure, a tale of abundance—of a "tidal wave" of love and care, of intimate and active networks of family and friends. But she is unflinchingly self-reflective about the layers of response this experience creates. There is a sense of guilt alongside gratitude, and more guilt in misery that is not at all allayed by expressions of fierce and self-sacrificing love.

The theology that happens here is similarly unsentimental. There is this agonizing conundrum: Why do drugs and prayer seem to work for her and not for her friend's beloved husband? There is this deep and sustained reality: "I ache, and God is silent. What do I do now?"

Again and again, Deanna states plainly, "there are no adequate answers for these questions." But her questions are themselves gifts of naming realities and mysteries on the hard edges of hope and the dark side of joy.

A hope and expectation of "cure" is in the vocabulary of modern science, and also in the vocabulary of the Bible. But it is something Deanna Thompson feels reluctant to pray for. What we experience with her instead is real, raw, ongoing work of healing that touches the whole of her life—her relationships, her body, and the very meaning of hope. She comes to acknowledge her "fractured-yet-graced life." She even introduces a piece of theology for our time: the Virtual Body of Christ.

No one knows how to have cancer, Deanna Thompson hears at one point and then learns the hard way. In the course of her treatment for Stage IV cancer, she is given advice about how to live while preparing to die. This book is a companion not merely for the illness of cancer but for that challenge, which ultimately defines all of our existence. All of our lives are fractured yet graced. This book is a gift as we make that discovery.

Krista Tippett

Preface

GETTING PAID TO TALK about God is a pretty sweet deal. As a religion professor, I spend my days talking—out loud and on paper—about the really big questions of life. My conversation partners, whether they are students, church members, friends, or family, are living those questions, sorting through inheritances, exploring the gaps, striving to be faithful to what they believe to be true. This profession of mine affords me the privilege of getting to talk about God in ways that are always informed by the questions, claims and wagers of others.

Then cancer came along and interrupted the conversation.

As an expert talker, I suddenly was no expert at all. A novice with a cancer story different from any other I knew. Breast cancer was the diagnosis, but my narrative didn't include finding a lump, removing a breast or losing any hair. A broken back triggered the stage IV cancer diagnosis and a lousy prognosis: five years out, eighty percent of those who have what I have are dead. My lack of expertise, unfamiliarity with the journey, and fear of what lay ahead conspired against me. Cancer left me tongue-tied, groping for words.

This is a story about cancer and what it steals from rich, full human lives. But the heart of this story is not really about cancer at all: it's about the real-life communion of saints and the incarnation of divine love that ushers salvation into the midst of the wretchedness. This is a story of amazing grace, mediated through prayers of children, hands of family, feet of friends, gifts of strangers. It's a story of acceptance of the grace that *is* rather than the grace that *could be*.

This story takes place in the Minnesota neighborhoods, hospital rooms, bedrooms, classrooms, and sanctuaries where I live, love, teach, worship, and pray. It is in those spaces—accompanied by those who incarnate the hands and feet of divine love—where I grieve what is lost and slowly embrace what is not. As words return and I learn to talk about cancer while talking about faith, the conversation pushes beyond the predictable parameters of prayer, the church, even hope in life after death.

Refracted through the lens of cancer, my life as wife, mother, daughter, sister, friend, and professor looks very different than it did before cancer. Refracted through the lens of cancer, faith looks different too.

Through the telling of this story of life and faith with stage IV cancer, I hope to offer what I wish I had had: a story about talking faith in the midst of cancer and talking cancer in light of faith; a way of speaking that resists conventional language about God's relationship to suffering, particularly in its cancerous form. The story that follows is no sentimental "God saved me from cancer" tale; instead it's an accounting of faith's faltering speech in the face of grim prognoses and brief glimpses of hope.

No doubt about it: cancer has changed virtually every aspect of my life. One thing that hasn't changed, however, is my understanding of myself as more sinner than saint. In public talk about cancer, there's a temptation to cloak cancer patients with a disease-induced righteousness. Or to suggest that those of us suffering from cancer possess a saint-like status that separates us from those who are cancer-free. But experience tells me that even though I've suffered much from cancer—even though I have undergone significant character adjustments because of the cancer—sainthood remains elusive, out of reach.

The fact that I'm still a sinner is precisely why I'm stuck on hope. As a person who never quite gets it right, I'm always hoping for more in this life—more chances to be gracious, kind, loving. Beyond these basic hopes, new hopes for this life have become important, too: hope for continued inactivity of the cancer in my body and in the bodies of so many others, for psychological and spiritual courage to live with this disease, for the gift of living long enough to see my daughters grow into adulthood.

In addition to hoping for more in this life, I also hope for more beyond. I hope that the promises of God are true: that there is more to life beyond this earthly one; and that in that life beyond there will be no more crying, no more dying, only light, only love, only joy.

My movement from fracture to hope has been possible only through the awe-inspiring support of family, friends, coworkers, neighbors, medical professionals, and church communities. My gratitude extends far and wide, but most especially to the following individuals and groups of persons who have made living with cancer possible:

- to the exceptional physicians, nurses, technicians, and staff at Abbott Northwestern Hospital, its Radiation Oncology clinic, the Twin Cities Spine Center, and Minnesota Oncology, especially Dr. Margaret MacRae and Dr. Amir Mehbod for their lifesaving care;

- to the compassionate, caring staff and congregations of Gloria Dei Lutheran Church in Saint Paul, Minnesota; Hope Lutheran Church in West Des Moines, Iowa; and other communities of faith that have held me in prayer—especially to Gloria Dei parish nurse Mary Jo Hallberg for her expert care and loving friendship;

- to the fabulous faculty, staff, students and administrators at Hamline University and in the Department of Religion, especially Jenny Keil, Mark Berkson, Kris Deffenbacher, and Mike Reynolds;

- to the wonderful attorneys and staff at Dorsey LLP and its Health Group, especially Raquel Smith;

- to those dear friends who have walked with and for me, especially Cindy Kaus, Char Hess and John Baldwin;

- to all those who lovingly—and secretly—stitched a quilt for us, especially Peggy Andrews, Jenny Keil, and Elaina Bleifield and families for their stunning work and friendship;

- to the community of parents from Horace Mann Elementary School, especially Eileen Moening and Kelly Trewartha, for the endless stream of meals and laundry service;

- to the teachers and administrators at Horace Mann Elementary and Capitol Hill Magnet School in Saint Paul, especially Kathy Ames, Amy Kordeum, and Doug Lewer for their attentive care of our daughters during an awful year in their lives;

- to our neighbors, especially the Polleis, Schoettlers, and Hanna-Kaplans for their steady gifts of food, snow shoveling, love and concern;

- to our friends near and far who have held us in prayer, sent notes, cards, jewelry, blankets, and blueberries, especially Lillian Daniel, Verity Jones, Kristen Looney, Karen Bastian, and Alzada Tipton for their friendship and special visits to St. Paul, and to Peter Nilsen-Goodin and Aaron Heley Lehman for their rock-solid support of Neal.

I am also indebted to those who read parts of this manuscript: Deborah Keenan, Mike Reynolds, John Baldwin, Maya Hanna, Rita Brock, Peggy Andrews, Lois Tverberg, Nicole Heley Lehman, Jenny Keil, Beth Gunderson, Michele Bassett, Dianne Oliver, Martin Copenhaver, Jim and Sonya Gindorff. Their feedback affirmed the importance of telling this story and deepened my ability to tell it. Special thanks also to Pam Fickenscher for the encouragement to begin writing, to Lillian Daniel for her guidance and inspiration throughout the writing process and to Mary (Joy) Philip for passing my proposal on to the publishers.

In this litany of gratitude, the best has been left for last. I would not have been able to hope for more without the support of my family: to my parents, Jackie and Merv Thompson, for their astounding love and care; to my parents-in-law, Erna and Glenn Peterson, for their abiding support and concern; to my brother, Noel, and sister-in-law, Ann, and family for their consistent care and for setting up the CaringBridge Site; to my sister- and brother-in-law, Naomi and David Tetzlaff and family for their support and guidance through the medical maze of hospitals, clinics, scans, and treatments; to my grandmother, aunts, uncles, and cousins for all their prayers and support.

At the heart of the fracture and the hope stand my strong and beautiful daughters, Linnea and Annika Thompson Peterson, and my incredible husband, Neal Peterson. To Linnea and Annika: I'm grateful beyond words for your resilience and your steady support of me, of your dad and one another. Know that my fierce love for each of you will never die.

Dear Neal, know that you are my life, my love, my all. May this book live on as a testimony to my never-ending love and gratitude for all that you have been, are, and will be for me.

one

Fractured

PEOPLE USED TO MARVEL—SOMETIMES with admiration, sometimes with envy—at my near-perfect life. I didn't discredit such observations. I knew I was fortunate. I'd married my college sweetheart, found a job teaching religion at a Minnesota university close to family, given birth to two beautiful daughters, and was surrounded by a tight network of support. I called it my 95 percent ideal life. A more spacious kitchen and fewer late-afternoon meetings and I'd be at least at 97 percent.

But during the summers, when we ate on our patio and work meetings came to a halt, my ideal life percentage closed in on a perfect score.

My love affair with life in general and summer in particular was going strong in 2008. In June I had boarded a plane to South Africa for a two-week travel seminar for college faculty.

I returned to Minnesota just long enough to readjust my internal clock before boarding another plane with my husband, daughters, and extended family for a two-week trek across Scandinavia. The eleven of us traveled from Stockholm to Bergen, spending time with relatives and tracing family roots to the farms and churches of Sweden and Norway. It was only August and this summer ranked high in the running for Best Summer Ever.

1

On a humid mid-August day I headed out to our neglected backyard gardens to thin the growing weeds. As I worked, crouched over my spade, I couldn't ignore the burning sensation in my lower back.

I had been dealing with lower back pain for much of the summer, pain I thought was related to weightlifting I'd been doing in an exercise class. The pain had camped out in my lower back, keeping a low profile but refusing to leave.

But the burning was new. When pain invited burning to set up camp, too, I decided it was time to evict them both.

Later that week I made an appointment at a near-by chiropractic clinic. I had never visited a chiropractor before; then again, I'd never had back pain before. Perhaps a few visits to the chiropractor would take care of my aching—and now burning—back.

Before meeting with the chiropractor, I filled out an extensive questionnaire about my pain. The visit that followed went well; after a brief examination, the chiropractor confirmed my back was out of alignment. She did some adjusting; my left side felt better. The chiropractor noted, however, that my right side wasn't cooperating. She recommended I return the following week for more adjustments.

My second appointment with the chiropractor wasn't as successful as the first. The chiropractor attempted again to adjust my right hip, but my body refused to cooperate. She tried several approaches, including raising the table and letting me drop several inches while she pushed on my right side. But there wasn't any adjustment like there'd been with my left side. After several unsuccessful attempts to get my back to cooperate, the chiropractor advised making another appointment so we could try again.

My sister- and brother-in-law are both physicians, and when they learned I had been to a chiropractor instead of a primary-care physician, they insisted I visit my primary-care clinic. Hesitant about more back adjustments, I decided to follow their advice and get another opinion about what was wrong with my back.

As a healthy forty-two year old who rarely visited a doctor, I did not have a primary-care doctor of my own, so I made an appointment with the first available physician. During the visit, the doctor confirmed significant swelling in my lower back. She suspected a pulled muscle. She prescribed pain medication for the swelling. I left the clinic, picked up the prescription, and hoped for the beginning of the end of my pain.

But all the pain meds did was make me groggy. The pain gave no indication of going away.

Frustrated, I talked to our church's parish nurse about my condition. After hearing of my failed attempts to get the pain treated, she told me, "You need to ask for an MRI. You need to find out what's going on with your back."

Knowing little about the medical world of tests, asking for an MRI hadn't occurred to me. Armed with this new information, I called the primary-care clinic, informing the nurse that the pain meds hadn't helped and that I needed an MRI. It took a bit of persuading to get the nurse to ask the doctor for an MRI without a follow-up visit, but after talking through the persistent nature of my pain, she put in the request with the doctor and an MRI was scheduled.

I have to admit I haven't always been the most cooperative patient. When I was a child, I was predisposed to sore throats and categorically opposed to throat cultures. I remember heading to the doctor with my mother when I was in grade school; she worked hard to bribe me into obediently subjecting myself to the impending throat culture.

But the bribe wasn't compelling enough to breed cooperation. Once In the examining room, I hid behind a chair and refused to get on the exam table. My next memory is of being held down on the table and the doctor prying open my mouth, cursing under his breath: "If you bite me, so help me God . . ."

But that was years ago. I was confident I had matured into a more agreeable, rule-following patient.

The problem was I had never had an MRI.

Thankfully the technician working the day of my MRI was a compassionate human being as well as a competent medical professional. She helped me lie down on the board that moves inside the machine. She asked whether or not I was claustrophobic.

"No," I replied proudly, recalling my recent descent into a South African cave to view ancient human remains while less adventurous colleagues had politely demurred, citing claustrophobia.

The MRI technician positioned the headphones on my ears, draped a blanket over my mid section, handed me the buzzer for emergency exit of the machine, and left the room to start the imaging.

I entered the machine with my eyes closed.

But I didn't keep them closed.

Peering out at the white curves of the machine just inches from my nose, I realized that I *was* claustrophobic, at least in MRI machines. I panicked and jammed my finger into the buzzer. The machine shut down and out I came. My heart raced and rather than running to hide behind a chair, I took the more adult route and began to cry.

The technician, a bit shocked at this reaction—especially after my confident assurance that I definitely was not claustrophobic—said, "Oh dear. You're OK, honey. Don't worry. We have some options on how to deal with this."

She reviewed my choices. Option one involved getting on my primary-care doctor's calendar, having her prescribe some Valium, driving to the pharmacy to pick it up, returning to the clinic, taking the Valium, having the MRI, and then finding someone to drive me home.

Sensing my hesitation over the first option, the technician continued: "Or we could turn you around and put you in the machine head first so that your head is closer to the opening on the other side."

I blinked back the tears. I'd try option number two.

Back into the MRI machine I went. Head first, eyes closed. The technician turned up the volume on the music flowing to my headphones. Forty-five minutes later, I had survived my first MRI.

The next day I received a call from the primary-care doctor. "We got the results of your MRI." She paused. "You have a fractured vertebra in your lower back."

A fractured spine, I repeated to myself. That's not what I had expected to hear.

The doctor continued, "I'd like you to see a spine specialist for treatment."

I took down the number for the spine clinic and made an appointment for the following week.

⌒

People often ask me whether learning about the fracture in my back sparked any premonition of what lay ahead.

Other than some annoying back pain, I felt great. I had no idea that my near-perfect life was beginning to slip away.

two

Diagnosis

THE FOLLOWING WEEK I met with a physician's assistant at a local spine clinic. A few x-rays and several health questionnaires later, the P.A. showed me pictures from my MRI and reviewed with me the fracture in my lower back. He informed me that he was ordering a variety of tests—a bone scan, a bone density test, and a few others—to better determine why I had a broken vertebra.

"It could be that you had a weak bone there. It could be a fluke; sometimes bones just break," he said.

I nodded in agreement. A few years before, my then-five-year-old fell while running through our kitchen. When my husband took her to the doctor, they found out that our daughter's upper arm was broken. An x-ray revealed a small hole in her bone that the doctor had insisted was a fluke. Occasionally this happens in bones, the doctor explained. He suggested that the break might even strengthen the bone when the hole fills in as the arm heals.

After hearing the story of my daughter's hole-in-the-bone, the P.A. nodded, agreeing that "fluke" was a distinct possibility.

"Typically, though," he added, "you should have fallen off a roof to cause a break like this."

I heard the warning and prepared for more tests. By the time my visit with the P.A. was over, I had a prescription for Vicodin,

6

appointment cards for several tests, and a scheduled fitting for a back brace at a nearby orthopedics clinic.

Even though I struggled for breath the first time the technician cinched my new brace across my torso—and had to loosen it in order to drive home, fearing I'd pass out—I quickly grew to appreciate my protective mid-section cocoon. Colleagues at work called it my plastic corset as they admired the way it wound tightly around my hips and breasts and the ease with which it could be camouflaged under my fall wardrobe.

The forced immobility of my back caused by the brace—as well as the Vicodin—eased the pain. I was relieved; a couple months of wearing the brace and I would be back to normal. My brace became a reliable friend, offering steady support without demanding much in return.

In mid-October, I headed downtown to the hospital for the scheduled tests, passing them all with flying colors. The bone scan highlighted the fractured vertebra but little else. The technician conducting the bone density test told me that my bones had the density of a woman in her early thirties. For someone approaching birthday number forty-two, that was heartening news.

After wearing the brace continuously for several weeks, the P.A. recommended I go without it for a few hours a day so my stomach muscles wouldn't atrophy. I did as I was told and my back felt stronger each day.

By mid-November, I had less than two weeks remaining in the brace-wearing time frame. My appointment with the P.A.—where I hoped to take the brace off for good—was scheduled for the Monday after Thanksgiving. I spent November counting the days until I would be granted permission to return to a brace-free life.

On the Wednesday before Thanksgiving I experienced more pain than usual getting myself up, dressed, and ready for the day. After dropping my daughter off at school, I drove to campus, parked my car in the lot, opened the door, and shifted my weight to my left leg as I stepped out of the car.

Pain shot through my leg and back, causing me to clutch the car door to keep from falling. I stood there, clinging to my car in the parking lot, attempting to breathe through the pain, wondering if I'd be able to walk the couple blocks to my office. Determined to get through this last day of teaching before the Thanksgiving break, I gingerly eased my weight back onto my legs and hobbled slowly to my office.

The pain persisted throughout the day. It continued through Thanksgiving festivities, worsening until I had trouble walking, sitting, getting up from a chair and lying down. I resorted to taking Vicodin during the day instead of only at night, which reduced the pain slightly but left me nauseous. I called the spine clinic for help, but they informed me I would have to wait for new prescriptions until I saw the P.A. the following Monday.

My November countdown was no longer for the discarding of my brace; instead I counted the hours until I could be prescribed non-nauseating pain medication for during the day.

For the rest of the holiday weekend, I lived on over-the-counter pain relievers and when the pain became too great, opted for less pain and more nausea with the Vicodin.

Driving proved difficult and painful, so my husband drove me to my Monday appointment at the spine clinic. As the P.A. observed the difficulty I had walking, sitting, and getting up, he prescribed some additional pain meds and recommended another MRI.

The following day, December 2, my forty-second birthday, I braved my second trip into the crypt-like imaging machine. No buzzer pushing needed this time; I went in headfirst.

The next day I received a call from the P.A. His voice carried a new grim quality. "A second vertebra has fractured," he stated. "That's not good news. When you're wearing a brace, your back should be healing, not fracturing further."

I was dumbfounded. Even though the pain was severe, it hadn't occurred to me that another vertebra could have fractured. The P.A. recommended I see a spine doctor. In talking to the scheduler at the spine clinic, however, I learned that the first available appointment with this new doctor was two weeks away.

This is the point at which having family members in the medical profession is a real bonus.

Throughout the fall, we had regularly updated my brother- and sister-in-law on my condition. We had shared with them the test results and the P.A.'s recommendations from each visit. Once we told my brother-in-law about the second fractured vertebra, though, he decided it was time to intervene. He set up a visit to a respected spine surgeon at his hospital.

The following Monday my husband, my MRI reports and I were in the spine surgeon's office, anxious to find out more.

The doctor examined my MRI pictures with us, pointing to what he said was fluid surrounding the two fractured vertebrae. "This fluid is a bit mysterious," he explained. "I'd like to have it biopsied. One in a thousand chances it's cancer, but it'd be nice to be sure."

He also took note of my struggles to get on and off of the examining table.

"You know, we could just admit you to the hospital, do the biopsy, and work to get your pain under control," the surgeon proposed.

But this was the last week of my university's fall semester. I had papers to grade. Our girls needed to get to all their activities. Even though the pain was mounting, hospitalization seemed a bit extreme. The surgeon ordered the biopsy for later that day and after heading home for a quick lunch, my husband and I returned for the outpatient procedure.

The biopsy procedure was a bigger ordeal than I had expected. Simply getting me to lie down on a gurney required the aid of several nurses. After the initial prep work, they flipped me onto my stomach, which again caused significant pain. By this time, tears stained my face.

The doctor performing the biopsy came into the biopsy room to meet with me. In response to the tears, he tried to be helpful: "It won't hurt; you'll be only vaguely conscious during the procedure."

But the pain—as excruciating as it was—was not my main worry.

"I'm worried about what you might find," I said in a quavering voice.

He had no response to that.

During the biopsy, my sister-in-law brought my daughters to the hospital. She and my daughters waited until the last possible moment before packing up for piano lessons. Just as they made their way toward the exit, the attendant wheeled me out in front of them.

I was shocked to see them and couldn't locate many words through the heavy sedation. Tears welled up in my younger daughter's eyes. My older daughter's face went pale. Tears filled my eyes again.

This was not a good start to the week.

My sister-in-law took the girls to piano and my husband took me home. I have little recollection of the next thirty-six hours. I stayed home, relied on painkillers and struggled to get through my students' final papers.

On Wednesday morning I sat grading at the dining room table when the phone rang. With significant effort, I rose to answer it.

"This is the spine surgeon," the voice said. "Is your husband home?"

"No," I told him, attempting to remain calm.

There was an awkward pause.

"Do you have the results of the biopsy?" I ventured.

"Yes I do," was all he said.

After another long pause, the surgeon spoke again in what seemed like a falsely calm way. "Could I get your husband's number?" I gave him the number and the call ended.

I returned to the dining room table and struggled to sit down, tears trickling down my cheeks.

I started to pray. "Please God, please God, please . . ." were the only words I could find.

I knew that the logical next step would have been to call my husband.

But I couldn't make myself get back up and go to the phone. The words refused to come. I strained to focus on the term papers in front of me as a sense of dread crept over me.

Twenty minutes later, the front door burst open.

I heard the sobs before I saw him enter the dining room. My husband, more undone than I had ever seen him, wrapped me in his arms and wailed, "I'm so sorry, D., you have breast cancer!"

three

Stage IV

WHAT?? BREAST CANCER?

Ok. Fine. I had breast cancer. My mom's survived breast cancer twice; two aunts and two cousins have had it as well. I had long anticipated breast cancer sometime in my future.

But the words *breast cancer* did not seem to tell me anything about my back. And I wanted to know what the hell was happening to my back.

I pushed back from my husband. "What does having breast cancer have to do with my fractured back?" I inquired calmly in the face of my husband's panic.

"The biopsy. . . shows the cancer. . . in your back . . . is breast cancer," my husband managed. "It's spread from your breast to your back," he relayed as tears dripped off his cheeks.

He went on to tell me—in words heavy with tears—that the surgeon had conferred with my doctor brother-in-law, telling him, "If she were my sister, I'd admit her to the hospital for a few days so that we can run all the necessary tests, set up radiation appointments and get her pain under control."

At this point, neither of us protested. It was time to go to the hospital.

My husband told me he had called both sets of parents on his drive home. I pictured my husband breaking the news to

12

them. This helped explain his near-hysterical reaction by the time he got home.

I also learned that my parents planned to pick up our daughters after school so we could go directly to the hospital. My husband and my parents had decided to wait and let us tell the girls about the cancer later that day.

As we threw things in a bag to take to the hospital, I focused on the disconcerting image of my parents spending the afternoon feigning normalcy while my girls wondered what was really going on. It didn't take long for me to decide I needed to go to the girls' schools myself before heading to the hospital. I needed to see them. I needed to put my arms around them and tell them I had cancer.

My husband called my parents and told them we were leaving to go to the girls' schools. My mom and dad gathered themselves together to meet us there.

In the back seat of the car, with my arms tight around their shoulders, I told each of my precious daughters I had cancer and that I was headed to the hospital for a few days.

My nine-year-old didn't know how to react, the news too big to take in.

My twelve-year-old managed an "Oh, no," before hugging me tightly back. "Grandma has had breast cancer, and she's doing great now," she said, as if to reassure herself. "That can happen to you, too."

I also talked to my parents before we said our good-byes. "I wish I could trade places with you," my mom whispered in a voice filled with sadness. But she remained strong and managed a smile, for she knew she needed to buoy herself for the coming hours with our girls.

My father, on the other hand, was a mess. He just held me and cried. As a parent myself, I imagined how horrible this day had become for them. I wished I could spare them the pain.

One last round of hugs and my husband and I departed for the hospital. I was numb; a surreal quality surrounded these first hours after the diagnosis. I was confused over how breast cancer was discovered in my back, and my husband—equally as ignorant of metastatic breast cancer as I was—did not have much more information than what he had already told me. Shocked and largely in the dark about what we were facing, we parked in the hospital ramp and found our way to my hospital room.

Minutes after we were admitted, the parish nurse from our church entered our room, sorrow in her eyes and a prayer shawl in her arms.

Seeing the shawl set my tears flowing again. Just months before, I had listened to a woman from our congregation talk about the comfort her prayer shawl from church had provided as she underwent treatment for breast cancer. During her presentation, I had fought back the tears, thankful that our church provided her with that tangible sign of our church's prayers, love, and concern for her.

And here I was, hours after being diagnosed myself, receiving my own prayer shawl from our church. I accepted it from our parish nurse, secured it around my shoulders and kept it within reach for what would become a three-day hospital stay.

In those first days after the diagnosis, I couldn't muster up the strength, the courage—the faith?—to pray myself. My constant clutching of the prayer shawl as I traversed the hospital floors—in a wheelchair, a movable bed, and even, a couple times, on foot—to and from tests offered access to this thing called prayer that suddenly proved elusive to me. The shawl offered tangible assurance that we weren't facing this life-shattering diagnosis alone; instead I was wrapped in the prayers of those who loved me.

That first evening in the hospital, we had two other important visitors. We met for the first time with the oncologist recruited to my case by my brother-in-law. Her calm and compassionate demeanor reassured both my husband and me that we were in competent, caring hands.

The oncologist told us that the biopsy showed I had estrogen-receptive metastatic cancer, which meant that it most likely started in the breast and spread to my spine. She admitted that there was a slim chance it was ovarian cancer, but breast cancer was far more likely. She conducted a breast exam on me but didn't detect a tumor. She then informed us that the following day would bring a battery of tests, including a mammogram, to try and locate the cancer's source. If they found a tumor, they'd biopsy it so we could get an official diagnosis. I also needed a CT scan to find out if the cancer lurked in places other than my spine.

Calmly, patiently, the oncologist answered our questions, patting my hand as she talked. When at last we ran out of questions, she said goodnight and told us we would see her again the following day.

The other visitor was our pastor, who arrived moments before the oncologist finally made it to our room. Our pastor waited until the oncologist had left. Then she prayed for us. That was a gift, because we were out of words, especially for prayer.

After our pastor left, my husband and I prepared for sleep, ready to end this dismal day. I considered it a small act of grace that my pain was finally under control. My exhaustion was also accompanied by a strange feeling of relief that came from knowing—however little we actually understood—what was wrong.

I slept better than I had in weeks.

❧

The next day began with the CT scan, which involved lots of drinking of dye and much pain-filled moving onto and off of examining boards.

The breast center was our next stop. With my last mammogram coming back clear just months before, I asked the technician whether all this cancer could have emerged since that late-August test. The technician looked doubtful. "Let's see what this mammogram shows," she said.

Mammogram completed, I was helped back into my traveling bed to wait for the results. Without much delay, the report came back that no tumor was found.

"But we think a tumor's there somewhere, so we're going to try an ultrasound," the technician said. When I asked what an ultrasound would show, the technician replied, "Ultrasounds have much higher magnification capabilities than mammograms. And since your breast tissue is so dense, the ultrasound may show something that the mammogram can't see."

So into another room I was wheeled and with the use of an ultrasound probe, it didn't take the technician long to spot what she suspected was a tumor. She left to fetch the radiologist. Less than a minute after arriving to look at the monitor, the radiologist confirmed the technician's suspicions and prepared for a biopsy. They biopsied the tumor on the breast and later that day we had confirmation that the tumor was, in fact, malignant.

It was official; I had stage IV breast cancer.

When I wasn't undergoing tests, I was back in my hospital room, which had become a hub of activity for medical professionals, family members, and a close friend from my university. Loved ones seemed to show up just as I was summoned to my next test. At one point, my brother, sister-in-law and friend spent almost two hours waiting in my room while I was wheeled from one test to another.

Their presence proved useful in more than simply a supportive way: it was during that time that the spine surgeon stopped by, and this threesome was able to gather more concrete information about stage IV cancer and how it works.

I learned later that the spine surgeon acknowledged the grave nature of my condition. He also admitted that if I had gone much longer without treating my back, the damage to the spine could have been permanent. Thankfully, the upcoming treatment would almost assuredly prevent paralysis or other long-lasting effects.

Back in my room that second afternoon in the hospital, a breast surgeon—the one who would likely remove the tumor in my breast—paid my husband and me a visit.

"I want to make sure you understand that you'll never hear the word 'cure.' There's no cure for what you have. Once it's in the bones, the best we can do is contain the cancer," was the surgeon's greeting.

Clearly he was intent on telling it like it was.

"You'll need to decide whether or not to have a lumpectomy, a single mastectomy, or a bilateral mastectomy. More and more women are choosing bilateral mastectomies. We'll meet again later to discuss those options."

Evidently he also had strong opinions and was not shy about sharing them.

"You'll also want to get tested for the BRCA I and BRCA II gene which will tell us whether or not your cancer is genetic."

At this point I decided I didn't like this surgeon.

When I wasn't lying in a hospital bed, suffering from a broken back and stage IV cancer, I was teaching college courses on Christian ethics and theology, where we studied and debated things like the ethics of genetic testing.

This surgeon was a black-and-white kind of guy in what I understand to be a world of gray. Even though most of my words seemed to have abandoned me since the diagnosis, this doctor's academic-debate-style approach spurred me on to play devil's advocate in response to his line of reasoning.

"Why would I need to know that kind of genetic information?" I challenged.

The surgeon brightened up, as if energized by the possibility of debate.

He acknowledged that the case for testing had its detractors, but he argued that finding out you have the gene leads many women to have a double mastectomy, even if they don't have any trace of breast cancer.

I reminded him I already had breast cancer.

With a smirk at my last remark, the surgeon emphasized again the value of genetic testing and assured me we would be able to continue this conversation when we met again. He shook our hands and headed out of the room.

Welcome to the world of cancer, I thought as I watched him go.

Another welcome to the world of cancer came later that day when we were paid a visit by the hospitalist—a physician who sees patients only in a hospital setting—colleague of my hospitalist-brother-in-law. She entered my room and sat down to talk with us about the results of my recent CT scan. She started listing off the places in addition to the spine where cancer appeared on the report: the hip, the tailbone, the pelvis. She listed close to dozen different bone locations in all.

But the hospitalist wasn't finished. She informed us that there were also indeterminate spots on the left lung, the ovaries and thyroid.

As the list of cancerous places grew my vocabulary seemed to shrink proportionately.

While my husband and I started to cry, the hospitalist drew a long breath, on the verge of losing composure herself.

After a long pause, the hospitalist asked if we had questions. If there were questions to ask, we didn't know what they were. Facing our bleary eyes one last time, the hospitalist told us how sorry she was and left the room.

That night my parents brought our daughters down for their first visit since I had been admitted to the hospital. I was thrilled to see them; at the same time, I was becoming aware of how bad this stage IV cancer business can be.

Rather than discussing the most recent reports, we talked about school, about who had stopped by with food and flowers, about my pain being under control, about what great care I was receiving from the nurses and other medical staff (I saved the part about the opinionated surgeon for another day).

As they prepared to leave, the oncologist appeared at the doorway. She warmly greeted each of our daughters and my parents, then sat down to talk about where we were at, this second day of my life as a stage IV cancer patient.

Aware that my family and I had heard enough bad news to last a few lifetimes, the oncologist turned our attention toward treatment: she was putting me on Tamoxifen right away, an anti-estrogen drug with a proven track record of arresting the spread of the estrogen-receptive cancer. She also informed us that the following day I'd be prepped for radiation on my hip and back, which would work to kill the cancer cells that were eating away my bones in that region and causing me such intense pain.

In response to questions about the cancer in the breast (indeed, all of us knew the breast cancer drill: when you get breast cancer, you have surgery, chemotherapy, and radiation on the breast), we got another lesson in how different stage IV breast cancer is from the other stages of breast cancer. Once the cancer has spread, the focus shifts from the breast to the other cancer locations. Our main concern now, the oncologist informed us, was the hip and the back. The Tamoxifen would hopefully slow the cancer's growth in the breast while radiation would hopefully halt the cancer that could paralyze me if left unattended.

Facing the palpable fear lurking within each member of my family, our oncologist concluded boldly, "And once we get you set up for radiation, you're free to go home. You will be home for Christmas and hopefully for many more Christmases to come."

The oncologist was quickly becoming a beacon of hope in what seemed an increasingly desperate situation.

∽

I spent the following day in the radiation wing. Technicians measured and marked my hips, back, and torso for the coming radiation sessions. I met with the radiation oncologist, who walked us through the next month of daily treatments.

Before we left radiation, we were visited by a nutritionist who prepped us on how to eat while dealing with the side effects of radiation. We left the radiation wing with a bag of sample nutritional supplements that would help us survive the coming weeks.

I later learned it typically takes several weeks to wade through the tests and meetings I underwent in three days. By Friday night, I was on my way home with the prayer shawl around my shoulders; a journal given by my friend filled with notes from our meetings with all types of medical personnel; a growing number of floral arrangements from family, colleagues, and friends; a small pharmacy of drugs; and an appointment to start radiation the following Tuesday.

I was a cancer patient with only an inkling of what lay ahead.

four

Grace amidst the Ruins

IN THE MIDST OF the suffering and grief cancer brings, ties binding me to others were cast in stark relief. While cancer has pushed away some in my life, the far greater reality has been the embrace of family, friends, colleagues, neighbors, even acquaintances who sojourn with me through the painful journey of life with stage IV cancer.

It's humbling to be on the receiving end of such extravagant love. I'm grateful beyond words. I'm also slightly guilt-ridden.

What did I do to deserve these gifts of grace?

What words can express my gratitude for such gifts?

Words remain elusive and I adjust to my new role as recipient of grace as cancer does its best to strip me bare.

My Husband

Ever since our earliest days of dating, my husband's love and devotion for me has been his top priority. At the same time, he's also known for taking the long view of love, life, and happiness.

Take our path together after engagement: we spent several years—both before and after marriage—attending graduate and law school in separate states. While these years apart caused me to doubt the wisdom of our partnership, my husband took the long view, patiently reviewing with me why we were together, why we had chosen to pursue graduate school simultaneously in different states, and how wonderful our future together would be. After five years of living apart, our two households finally converged into one, just in time to welcome into our lives our first baby girl and my first full-time teaching position.

As our family grew and the demands of our jobs increased, my husband again took the long view. While I tend to immerse myself in the present to the point of ignoring the long view, my husband steadfastly, consistently, denies himself in the present for anticipated rewards in the future. From the day he began working as a lawyer in his mid-twenties he has planned to retire in his fifties and devote more time to his loves: me, our girls, our extended family, and golf.

Then cancer came along and struck a devastating blow to my husband's long view of life. I watched as his worldview fell to the floor in big, jagged pieces. What he had long believed to be true— that his life of delayed gratification would lead to a future full of time with the loves of his life—was put in serious doubt by my diagnosis. Even as the oncologist expressed hope for many more Christmases to come, it did not take us long to put our hands on the statistics for stage IV breast cancer: five years out from diagnosis, eighty percent of people who have what I have are dead.

Faced with the news of stage IV cancer, my husband stumbled, fell, and struggled mightily to get up.

While I have often wished my husband would live more fully in the present, since the diagnosis I have longed to replace the new worldview he's been forced to embrace with his old one.

But embrace this new reality he has, and I've been gifted in new ways by his embodiment of the scripture passage read at our wedding years some eighteen years before: "Where you go, I will go; where you lodge, I will lodge; your people shall be my people, and your God my God" (Ruth 1:16). From his detailed notetaking during doctor appointments to his constant presence during my days in the hospital to his cleaning up the vomit following radiation and other treatments, my husband demonstrates—even in the midst of the extraordinary challenges of our new reality—that he will go wherever I go, even to the depths of sadness, despair, and grief.

His love for me is like God's love for me: I didn't earn it, I often don't deserve it, but I can be grateful, to God and to him, for his continued, consistent presence in this journey.

Our Daughters

The fall before the diagnosis, as we worked through a disagreement, my older daughter looked up at me and said, with a hint of condescension in her voice, "Perhaps we should get to know each other better."

With these words, my daughter officially entered adolescence. Her underlying message, it seemed to me, was that I didn't know her as well as I should and I needed to work harder to understand the complicated person she knew herself to be.

This daughter who hibernates in her room with a book or a pencil in hand, only venturing out to eat, visit the bathroom, or use the computer, was saying to her always-inquisitive mother that I needed to try harder at this relationship?

My cancer diagnosis certainly changed my daughter's perspective; but it did so, especially at first, by robbing her of an adolescent's prerogative to be self-absorbed. In a matter of days, my eldest was thrust not only from the center of her own world but from ours as well. She began to cope instinctually, by asking questions, hoping the answers would give her a keener sense of what it was that displaced her position in the world. She and I were comfortable with our roles in these discussions: she inquired and I attempted to offer satisfactory answers.

But other conversations were less predictable. On a night shortly after the diagnosis, my daughter crept into my bedroom just as I was drifting off to sleep.

"Mom, can I talk to you?" she whispered.

My body craved sleep but I sensed this might be one of those "getting to know each other better" moments I needed to have more of. I slowly moved over and invited her into the bed.

She crawled under the covers and began to tell me about problems with a friend from school who badgered her about whether or not she *liked* a boy. We talked a few minutes about her friend's persistent questioning. Then I took a risk and forged ahead into some new territory.

"So *do* you like anyone?" I asked, clueless of what the response might be.

Slowly she nodded her head up and down. I forged ahead delicately, looking for signs that I had overstepped my bounds.

But my daughter was in a divulging mood and after close to an hour-and-a-half of conversation, I hugged my daughter tightly and she headed off to bed.

This late-night conversation became the first of many conversations with my daughter about all aspects of her life as an almost-thirteen year old. One unexpected gift of being confined to the house for several months was the opportunity for the two of us to talk. Hearing her walk in the front door was one of the highlights of my day. Whether conscious or not, my daughter seemed to realize not only that she needed me, but also that I needed her in this post-diagnosis life. Talking time with her has been one of the most precious gifts of my post-diagnosis life.

While my older daughter delights in long debates and analytical conversations, my younger daughter has scant interest in such things. At our all-female family weeknight dinners (my husband eats later after he's home from work), my younger daughter permits the academic conversations between her sister and myself to continue only so long before she pushes her hair back, sighs dramatically, and asks, "Can we *please* talk about something else?" She gives us that *How-did-I-get-put-in-this-family?* look, and her sister and I back off, moving on to lighter topics.

My younger daughter's insistence on changing the subject only intensified after the cancer diagnosis. While my husband worried she didn't have sufficient information about the realities of stage IV breast cancer, I hesitated to push more information at her. She already had to live with this new cancer diagnosis every minute of every day. Did she need really to talk about it too?

While my youngest is not passionate about long conversations, she's passionate about spreading joy whenever and wherever she can.

Several years ago, the mother of a child suffering with leukemia told me that my daughter was one of the only classmates who "got" her daughter's illness. She described how my daughter stayed with her daughter during the times when most first graders backed away, unsure of how to act.

To some extent, I suppose that my daughter's caring disposition has been shaped by the family and friends who love her. At the same time, much of it seems innate.

Before the diagnosis, when she and I snuggled together before she was off to sleep, she would thank me for dinner, for picking her up from here or there, for being her mom.

What had I done to deserve such sweet whispers of grace? Not enough, that's for sure. My daughter's gifted with a compassionate soul and she shares that gift liberally with any and all who know her.

And after the diagnosis, my youngest focused an inordinate amount of her compassionate care on me. She seemed to know instinctively when I needed companionship or support.

During one particularly bad winter afternoon, my daughter, armed with a book we had started to read together in the fall, crawled into bed with me and read out loud for over two hours. In life before cancer, she would typically read a chapter or two and then hand the book over to me, insisting I read the rest. But there she lay, snuggled next to me in bed, reading her heart out all afternoon. This subtle display of love nourished me for months to come.

My Parents

After years of attempting to retire "up north" next to a rural Minnesota lake, my parents admitted defeat and bought a place in the Twin Cities. My mom's desire to be involved in the lives of her five grandchildren coupled with my dad's dislike of up-north pastimes (fishing, hunting, snowmobiling, and reveling in the rural character of it all) led them to buy a house a few miles from me and my brother's family. With my brother and his wife working full time as well, both families benefitted greatly from my parents' move. We acquired built-in babysitters, chauffeurs to weekly activities, even a dinner-fairy who delivers hot meals during busy times. My mother, who lost both her parents before the age of thirty, has committed herself to being there for her own children and grandchildren as long as she's able.

Add my mother's life-changing experience of breast cancer—not once, but twice—to her fierce dedication to her children and you're left with volumes of care for her daughter, the cancer patient. In the months after the diagnosis, she was at our house almost every day, preparing dinner, rubbing my feet, holding my hand. As a cancer survivor herself, she anticipated my level of fatigue or the few foods I'd be able to ingest after radiation before I'd recognize these realities myself. I wish breast cancer wasn't a point of connection for the two of us, but that's the reality; and my burden of grief, pain, and despair has been lightened significantly through her and my father's support.

In addition to their support of me, my parents also provided a reliable presence for our girls. My parents virtually moved in, taking over most aspects of the girls' weekly schedules, driving them across the city for music or dance, assisting them with daily homework and other school projects, keeping them company during the long stretches of appointments and hospital stays. Life post-diagnosis would have been much more difficult—and more lonely—without their constant care.

His Parents

Among their many interests in life, my in-laws are passionate about all things home and garden. In the dozen years of owning our own home, they have shared this passion—and skill—with us. They put up the wallpaper that dons our walls, designed our gardens, and hand-selected our plants, planting many of them themselves.

After my hospitalization, my in-laws drove down from their home in Duluth and did what they do best: took care of our home. They purchased holiday wreaths for our entryway, dug Christmas decorations out of the basement and made the house look like Christmas, even though none of us felt much like celebrating.

Early in the new year, my mother- and father-in-law would come and stay with us again, putting away the Christmas decorations, taking me to radiation treatments, spending time with the girls. They filled needs wherever they noticed needs to be filled, working from morning until evening on the days they were here. From their home in Duluth, they kept in frequent contact with my husband, providing much-needed support for him in his new role as primary caretaker for his spouse.

Our Siblings

Even though my brother and I live just twenty minutes apart, we often go months without seeing each other's families. Our lives are full of jobs and kids' activities, which can leave little time for getting together. But from the day of the diagnosis on, my brother and his wife made themselves available to care for and be with my family and me. From spending hours in the hospital, to my sister-in-law's day of cleaning our house, to their prayers as a family for us, my brother and his family have been a strong presence in a bleak time. Perhaps the most significant gift, though, was my brother's creation of a CaringBridge site for me, an internet site designed to update family and friends of those with serious illness.

My sister-in-law and her husband live just minutes from our house as well. Their help negotiating the maze of medical offices—from the spine center to oncology, radiation, the breast center, and nuclear medicine—has been tremendous. Having my brother-in-law on staff at the hospital provided us with a second set of eyes and ears regarding my condition. Their constant willingness to review and explain what this test revealed and the purpose of that scan made the journey into this foreign world of medicine a bit less frightening. Their children's many cards to their auntie also made hospital rooms a less daunting place to be.

Our Community

Since moving back to Minnesota when our eldest daughter was just five weeks old, my husband and I have each worked in the same job for the past fifteen years. We both have invested serious time and energy into our workplaces; it's not surprising, then, that our workplaces responded quickly to my diagnosis with expressions of concern and offers of care.

But the level of support, concern, and help was far beyond what we could have imagined. We were simply, utterly overwhelmed.

Within days of the diagnosis my husband's secretary and colleagues had organized a month's worth of meals for our family. Each day my husband made it to work, he would return with elaborately prepared dishes made by someone in his office.

A week after the diagnosis, friends and colleagues at my university held a prayer service in my honor. The service was held in the morning; by early afternoon, I was hearing reports about the several dozen colleagues who had gathered in the chapel on my behalf.

All the stories included reference to a prayer given by one friend in particular, the one who had spent time with my family in the hospital the week before. This friend is the sister I never had; in fact, we look so much alike that we regularly get mistaken for the other. In the dozen years we have worked together at the university, I have received congratulations for her tenure decision; she has accepted praise for my book; even our university president once greeted me by my friend's name. These occurrences of mistaken identity humor us; they aso stand as a witness to our sister-like friendship.

One colleague who called to tell me about the service described my friend's prayer. "It's clear she loves you dearly," he said. I smiled amidst the tears. An even wider network of colleagues were learning of the fierce closeness I shared with this friend.

Later my friend shared with me the prayer she wrote for the university service, an anguished cry to God that put into words much of we could not yet say:

> Why Lord, why? We do not understand. None of this makes sense. But we believe that you love Deanna even more than we love Deanna, so we lean on your promises.
>
> You say do not worry about anything, bring everything to you in prayer, so we pray. We pray for no more pain. We pray that the radiation will work quickly and Deanna's back will heal. No more pain, Lord.
>
> We pray for Deanna's husband, Lord. Help him be strong, help him live one day at a time, help him not worry about the future and not to get ahead of himself.
>
> We pray for their daughters. Lord, be close to them. Comfort them. Help them help their mom.
>
> We ask that you work in a mighty way Lord—heal Deanna—take the cancer away. Her friends need her. Her family needs her. Our university needs her.
>
> We believe that you hear us when we pray Lord—help us be strong; help us help Deanna.
>
> It is the deepest cry of my heart that Deanna would be healed Lord. Heal her. Heal us. Help me in my unbelief.

The prayers of my friend—along with the prayers and words of our family, friends, and so many others—formed a tight circle of embrace into which we fell.

The circle of embrace widened exponentially in those first weeks through the CaringBridge site set up by my brother. Dozens of messages were posted each day.

A strange sense of comfort came in reading the many expressions of shock and sadness. One friend recently done with chemotherapy wrote, "This news stinks." A colleague's message began, "We're sick at heart."

Knowing the news stunned others helped us cope with our own shock and our own inability to give voice to the thoughts and emotions. So many who are dear to us sent words of comfort and we drew strength from each one.

One professor-friend of mine captured the limits of language to express the trauma caused by cancer's deep invasion into our lives. He also illuminated the power of a site such as CaringBridge to enable collective responses to and engagement with the most awful events of our lives:

> We all spend much of our lives differentiating the somewhat good, the mediocre, and the somewhat bad. The words for such things come easily. But the horrendous initially strikes us dumb. When we throw words at it, hoping to defend ourselves, the words fall flat.
>
> It is the same at the other end of the spectrum. The sacred ties our tongues. Only true poetry can give voice to the emotions the sacred elicits. But no words, however deeply felt or carefully chosen, can do the topic justice.
>
> This much, however, is clear. The two ends of the spectrum are linked. If we are right to regard some things as horrendous, and to respond to them initially with shock, that must be because whatever those things attack is rightly regarded with reverence and love. There is some consolation in that thought, because it means that we do live among others worth cherishing. Our shock, on reflection, is a revelation of value. It teaches us what we actually care about and should care about.
>
> The shock registered in so many of these Guestbook entries requires expression. It helps us, your friends, to put

in words, however feebly, the love on which the shock rests. Nothing would be gained, for you or for us, by tarrying in the shock. We must somehow move on. You are surely already doing so, and you will have to be patient while our emotions catch up. But as we do move on, into this next phase, you need to know, and we need to say, that we are thinking of you, and pulling for you, every day.

In the days after it was posted, I read and reread my friend's message. He was dead on: words to describe both the grief and the grace seemed consistently out of reach. That he gave voice to the excruciatingly beautiful connections between the sorrow and the grace helped me begin to accept my role as recipient of the lavish grace that continued to come our way.

The love and support we experienced extended far beyond the CaringBridge site to in-person care of friends and neighbors in the midst of those dark December days.

Close friends visited the house soon after I came home from the hospital, bearing gifts of books, jewelry, ginger ale, and coffeecake. They came for short, focused spurts of time, creating cleaning or sorting or errand-running tasks for themselves. Our Christmas cards even went out earlier than in the past ten years running; all because of the help friends offered.

Childhood friends of my husband gathered at our house the Saturday before Christmas to make and serve a pancake breakfast. The house filled with bright voices and even laughter, a welcome sound.

Families of my daughters' friends stopped by and brought food, tea, and gifts for the girls. One family took our girls Christmas shopping. Before long, parents from my younger daughter's school set up a web-calendar on the "What Friends Do" website, coordinating laundry and dinner duties for us from January to April. Families we knew well—such as the family of my daughter's friend who had leukemia, who had since become a healthy, happy fourth grader—and families from school we barely knew started picking up our laundry and bringing us dinner. Friends of my brother sent a day pass for downhill skiing for our daughters. A friend from work and a teenaged neighbor knit me scarves.

Neighbors came bearing cookies, muffins, and other comfort food. When snow fell—as it frequently does during Minnesota winters—they arrived with shovels and snow blowers, clearing our driveway and sidewalk. Amidst the snow, delivery trucks brought flowers daily to our door for what seemed like weeks. Our house became an oasis of blooming plants, the brightly-colored flowers bursting forth like little signs of hope in every room of the house.

While no one or no thing could alleviate the pain, the grief, or disorientation cancer brought to our lives, each of these persons and each of these gifts ushered glimpses of grace into the Advent darkness. I had cancer and had it bad. But I was also bound to individuals and communities whose love and care overwhelmed me, and without which I may not have survived.

five

Losing Our Grip

DESPITE THE TIDAL WAVE of support, readjustment to life after hospitalization proved frustratingly difficult. Worst of all was the ongoing, debilitating pain. At home I had a house full of loved ones willing to help me get up, sit down, climb stairs, and lay down; but managing the pain simply didn't happen at home as well as it had in the hospital. We all had to learn, through painful trial and error, how to help me navigate life back at home.

The oncologist and radiation oncologist both insisted that it could be as few as four or five radiation treatments before the pain in my back would decrease exponentially. I was desperate for the pain to ease and set my sights on the salvific power of radiation.

After the weekend at home, my husband took me back to the hospital Monday evening for my first treatment. Getting on and off the radiation bed was once again the most challenging part of the appointment, requiring the help of my husband plus three radiation technicians.

Once I was finally positioned correctly on the radiation table, all my helpers exited the room. I lay motionless as the machines radiated my spine and hip from above and below. I fought back tears, feeling exposed and alone amidst the buzzing and the clicking.

Before we left, the nurses gave us a prescription for anti-nausea medication. My husband and I returned home, ate a bit of dinner, and hoped for a quiet rest of the evening.

A quiet evening was not to be. The nausea came on quickly and unexpectedly, leaving me vomiting and crying out due to the excruciating pain caused by the heaving. Despite my heaving and my tears, my nine-year-old remained by my side, softly rubbing my back, trying to help make it better. My husband got on the phone and recruited a neighbor to pick up the anti-nausea meds we were prescribed just a few hours before. Our neighbor arrived quickly with the medication and I took it immediately. By that time, however, there was nothing left to keep down.

After several days of the radiation-throwing-up routine, I was told to take the anti-nausea medicine before—as well as after—treatment. This simple suggestion proved helpful. Food was still largely unappealing, but I no longer lost the contents of my stomach after every treatment.

As predicted, the pain in my back and hip began to recede. I was able to get on and off the radiation table with assistance from my husband and only one other assistant. I moved well enough to start walking with my husband at the mall, which is where you walk when it's winter in Minnesota and you have a broken back.

The week of Christmas—my second week of treatment—began with an atypical Sunday morning treatment, as the radiation clinic worked to fit in four days of treatment for their patients before the long Christmas weekend. On December 23, I had my "regular" 6:30 p.m. radiation treatment. At 6:30 a.m. on Christmas Eve morning we returned for a fourth treatment before the clinic closed early for the holidays. My husband and I, thankful for the holiday reprieve from the emotional and physical toll of radiation, headed to the local mall for a celebratory lap before returning home to enjoy the Christmas weekend with our family.

Later that afternoon, we drove to my parents' home to spend Christmas Eve with my parents and my brother's family. After the trauma of the past two weeks, the festive dinner, present opening, and the play performed by my daughters and their cousins were welcome respites from the world of cancer that had invaded our lives.

My husband, daughters, and I even made it to church for the Christmas Eve service. It was emotional return for me, to be back among the people who had wrapped me in my prayer shawl. We slipped in to the balcony as the service began and ducked out early to avoid most of the greetings, embraces, and conversations I was not yet able to face.

The force of the compressed radiation treatments began to catch up with me on Christmas Day. I threw up in the morning, then stabilized enough to return to my parents' home for a gathering of extended family. We were grateful to spend the day with loved ones. Aunts and uncles and cousins all gave me extra-long hugs, and there were special gifts—such as a "recovery" calendar filled with photos of me and other family members—and again we aspired to be festive and enjoy this grand holiday of our religion and our culture.

But my grandma would have none of it. Approaching ninety years old and traveling rarely, this was the first time we had seen each other since the diagnosis. I was told that she cried for two days after she heard the news; and at this family Christmas gathering, Grandma didn't hide her sorrow. She sat next to me and cried. As the tears fell, she kept her hand on my knee, asking questions about my back, my pain, my treatment.

A photograph from that day shows my grandma sitting next to my daughter and me on the couch, surrounded by the sparkling Christmas decorations of my parents' home. My daughter and I both are smiling, but Grandma is frowning, eyes red and puffy. The photo testifies to the line we all walked between striving for normalcy in the midst of gut-wrenching grief and sadness.

Unfortunately for me, Christmas evening brought more nausea and vomiting. The two weeks of treatment caught up with me with violent, cumulative force.

Saturday, the day after Christmas, I threw up every time I tried to eat. By evening, I opted for a liquid diet. Sunday I began throwing up after each sip of liquid.

I had never felt so sick in my life.

At five a.m. Monday morning, after struggling to the bathroom and moaning as I crawled back into bed again, my nine-year-old tiptoed into our bedroom.

"Can I rub your feet, Mom? I can't sleep, and I want to rub your feet."

I slowly made room for her on the end of the bed. She gently stroked my feet. After a few minutes, she covered my legs with the covers, gave me a hug, and returned to bed.

The panic momentarily subsided.

But as the morning light began to illumine the bedroom, I turned to my husband who lay next to me, exhausted and immobilized by fear and grief, and insisted: "Call the radiation clinic. Tell them I need to be admitted to the hospital."

He dialed the number and the radiation receptionist told us to come in early before my scheduled mid-morning appointment. My parents appeared at our door, my dad staying with the girls and my mom accompanying my husband and me to the hospital.

It didn't take long for the radiation nurses to send me to the ER. An ER doctor ordered fluids and soon I was meeting another hospitalist-colleague of my brother-in-law.

This hospitalist sat down and reviewed with us the last two weeks. He expressed sympathy for what I had been through. Then he looked at me directly and said, "I hope you know that none of this is your fault. You didn't do anything to cause what's happening to you."

Tears filled my eyes; the doctor's face grew blurry.

But his words were in focus: "What we need to do now is get fluids and nutrients back in you; we also need to figure out why you've been throwing up so much. It could be the radiation treatment is too strong for your body to withstand—after all, the radiation to your back comes really close to your stomach and intestines. But it could be you have some problem with your throat. We'll need to check that out, too. "

The hospitalist took a breath, allowing us space to take in what he'd just said. "We'll figure it out, and get you back to eating and drinking and feeling better." Before he left, he patted my leg as he told us that I'd be moved shortly to a hospital room, where I would stay until my condition turned around and headed in the right direction.

This hospital stay lasted six days, twice as long as the first visit earlier in the month. Our girls spent the rest of Christmas break living out of suitcases at my parents' and my sister-in-law's homes. My husband stayed with me in the hospital, sleeping on a makeshift bed wheeled into my room each night.

My husband and I spent a bleak New Year's Eve in the hospital room trying to find words to fill a conversation about what he'd do if I died.

Tearfully we decided where I'd be buried. Then we tried out words for the headstone. Toward the end of the conversation, I managed a few sentences about my hope that he would eventually find someone else to love.

"But I don't want to love anyone else," my husband whispered, words thick with grief. "You're the only one . . ."

As my husband fought back tears, I sensed we were out of words. I kissed his hand, hoping that the new year would bring us, among other things, new words.

Later that evening, as I attempted to sleep, my husband sat down at the computer by the nurse's station and summoned up more words for his only entry on CaringBridge. He knew that hundreds of people anxiously awaited word on my condition and that I wasn't well enough to be posting any time soon.

After updating readers on my re-hospitalization, my husband ended his post with these words,

> "In you, Lord, I put my trust . . . Be my strong refuge, to which I may resort continually." Psalm 71:1, 3. During these challenging days, we have resorted continually to

our God for strength and refuge. We give God thanks for the medical team caring for Deanna and for all of you for holding our family up in prayer. Our spirits are lifted by the thoughts, prayers, acts of kindness and expressions of support from all of you. They are all good medicine for our souls.

In the midst of this bleak time, my husband and I were sustained by the prayers, concern, and care of so many.

Most unexpected was the deep compassion displayed by physicians, technicians, and nurses. My oncologist visited daily; one nurse from my hospitalization three weeks earlier learned we were back and found time to visit my hospital room. She told me that after caring for me the first night of my diagnosis, I'd been in her prayers ever since.

"It's so unfair," the nurse said, "you're so young. You have a family who needs you. You seem so full of life."

I smiled sadly. *It is so unfair.* But the fact that the nurse who cared for me for a few hours had been praying for me dampened the despair a bit.

Time to despair was also kept to a minimum by the number of tests and doctor meetings scheduled each day. Shortly after being admitted, I had a PICC line—a long thin tube inserted into the peripheral vein—put in my upper arm. While the forty-five-minute process of getting the long tube threaded through my upper body was unnerving, the benefits of the PICC line were instantaneous and significant: no more painful, aborted attempts to find adequate veins in my hands and arms. I was hooked up to fluids and given my pain medication and anti-nausea drugs all through this wonderful little lifeline.

Determining the cause of all my throwing up was the other issue that demanded immediate attention. I was scheduled for an endoscopy, a procedure that slides a camera down the throat in order to view the insides of the esophagus and stomach.

As someone with a history of violent resistance to throat cultures, I was terrified by the descriptions of this particular test.

Doctors and nurses explained what would happen and *You'll be awake* and *You need to resist gagging* was all that stuck with me.

Thankfully the endoscopy went smoothly and quickly, the sedative so effective that after it was over I asked when it would begin. Only after the procedure did I realize that they were concerned about the possibility of throat or esophageal cancer as the cause of the constant vomiting. Thankfully the report came back clear. With a good report from the endoscopy, it was time to revisit the radiation doses.

My oncologist conferred with the radiation oncologist and they decided to reduce the intensity of the treatment to my back and to halt treatment on the hip altogether. They believed the radiation to the hip most likely caused the incessant vomiting. They explained to us that I had been receiving the highest radiation doses possible due to severity of the cancer in my vertebrae and hip. They were hopeful that the two weeks of completed treatments to my hip would have a lasting effect of killing most or all the cancer in that area.

Equipped with this new plan, I was wheeled back down to radiation oncology for repositioning, which entailed getting new black marker dots on my stomach. Shortly thereafter, I resumed radiation treatment.

After several days of IV fluids, I began drinking "clear liquids," working up to "full liquids" a few days later. At last, after more than a week without solid food, I started eating again. I was also sleeping better and on a radiation regimen that wasn't killing me.

Things were looking up.

After six days of hospital life, I was able to imagine leaving this cocoon of care and returning home.

We arrived home late Saturday night, my parents keeping the girls a final night to give us some time to settle in and to be together without the constant interruption of hospital life. Shortly after my parents brought our girls home the next morning, my nine-year-old asked to write the CaringBridge entry that went out to family and friends:

> My mom got out of the hospital last night. I was thrilled. We can finally be together as a family again. She is doing o.k. She ate a little breakfast of coffee cake and a couple bites of oatmeal. A big thank you to my grandparents and my aunt and uncle (and cousins) for having my sister and me stay with them while mom and dad were in the hospital.

I was ecstatic to be with my daughters again. We spent the day catching up on their adventures with grandparents, aunts, uncles, and cousins. The girls read out loud to me as we snuggled together. We ended the day with family prayers on our bed, grateful beyond measure for the support of family, friends, coworkers, teachers, and neighbors.

The words of thanksgiving from my daughters and my husband gave me hope that this might be the beginning of a new normal for us, for days free of the traumatic drama that had filled our lives over the past three weeks.

six

Take this Cancer from Me

BACK IN MY 95 percent ideal life, I spent most of my time outside the house.

I would walk my younger daughter to school each weekday morning, head to work at the university, leave campus in the late afternoon to pick up the girls for piano lessons, dance, or church. Weekends were spent at school functions, social events, family gatherings, and church.

Then cancer came along and put a stop to my outside-the-house life.

For the first two months of life with cancer, I was home or at the hospital, seeing only the family, friends, and neighbors who came to visit. My husband took over many of my daily tasks, such as walking our daughter to school each morning. During these early days, he would return crying, having talked with concerned parents and teachers about how I—we—were doing.

My husband and daughters attended church without me. The three of them would return after a Sunday service, and in response to my questions about the morning, my girls would tell me that their dad cried all the way through the service—*again.*

I slowly realized that while I struggled to get beyond the confines of my bedroom, my girls and especially my husband had become the public face of our journey with cancer, and that role had taken its toll.

Meanwhile radiation treatment continued into January. As expected, it siphoned off most of my energy and stamina. But the doctors' prediction of reduced back pain slowly became reality. It no longer took half a dozen hands to get me on and off the radiation table. I cut back on pain medication. It appeared radiation was killing the cancer cells and halting the destruction of my spine.

But it was also clear that the cancer cells had destroyed much of my two vertebrae, and as my pain receded, the fractured vertebrae compressed further, causing bones to protrude behind the skin of my lower back. The protrusions became so pronounced that the radiation technicians cut a hole in the back of my brace to prevent further damage to the skin already made sensitive by radiation.

This protrusion also led us back to the spine surgeon, who recommended vertebroplasty—a procedure that injects a cement mixture into weakened vertebrae to help strengthen the bone and reduce pain. My husband and I quickly agreed to this plan and set up the vertebroplasty for later that month.

In addition to daily radiation treatments, my other January task was to resign from my life.

Shortly after the diagnosis, my departmental colleagues stepped in and hired an adjunct professor to take over my January-term course. I handed over departmental chairing responsibilities to a colleague. I resigned from our university faculty council, from the search committee for a new vice president, from chairing our university diversity committee.

Beyond the university, I resigned my post as chair of a task force on the future of the profession for our national society of religion scholars; I also stepped down from the position of director of our professional society's regional chapter, handing over duties for the spring meeting to the director-elect.

The most painful letter of resignation I sent was to the organizer of the first-ever conference on Martin Luther and feminism, scheduled for later that month. Describing my academic interest in Luther and feminist theology would require another book (which thankfully I've already written); but suffice it to say, I anticipated this conference to be the most exciting event of my scholarly career thus far. Even though I desperately wanted to attend, I was all-too-aware that traveling to Chicago to give a lecture or participate in panel discussions was outside the realm of possibility.

Sending that letter brought me to a new low.

Still, I wasn't quite done resigning. I backed out of my part in leading a couples' retreat for our church. Then came the cancelling of the church confirmation and adult forums I was scheduled to lead, along with the art-appreciation sessions at my daughter's school. By the end of the month, my life as a cancer patient bore no resemblance to my 95 percent ideal life.

In fact, I scarcely recognized it as my life.

The only scheduled commitment from which I did not resign was teaching my Introduction to Theology course during spring semester. Due to my heavy responsibilities beyond the classroom, I had created the ideal spring teaching schedule for myself: one introductory-level course, in my area of expertise, meeting two mornings per week.

As radiation continued to reduce the pain, I grew more confident that I could handle this one class. I wrote on CaringBridge about my process of discernment regarding teaching in the spring, which a number of colleagues, friends, and family members had discouraged me from doing:

> Many of you have asked whether or not I will be teaching this spring. At this point, I'm inclined to do it. Perhaps some of you saw the article on Patrick Swayze, who's undergoing chemotherapy for cancer while working twelve-hour days for his new television series. "Of course I'm going through

hell," was his response to a reporter's question about how he's fairing.

Mr. Swayze and I have different approaches to living with cancer. Simply put, I have no desire to "go through hell." Landing in the hospital for a week was a little bit of hell, and I likely have more hell to go through before I'm through with this journey. But actively creating the conditions of hell?

No thanks.

What I realized after reading about Patrick Swayze was that I have no desire to be a martyr with respect to this cancer business. I have no intention of trying to keep up the pre-cancer pace to prove to others that cancer hasn't beaten me.

A few days after I posted this entry, I decided to teach my spring course, hoping it wasn't foolish to try and resist cancer's *total* claim of my life. Our new department chair reluctantly agreed to let me teach, even as he expressed concern about my stamina. By late January I had pulled out the syllabus from last year's theology course, changing only the meeting and due dates to make it as simple as possible for me to teach.

Toward the end of the month, I headed to the hospital for my final radiation treatment. As I sat up by myself after the treatment, I was greeted with cheers and hugs from the radiation technicians and nurses. They presented me with a certificate of graduation from radiation signed by each of them.

After saying our goodbyes to the compassionate staff in radiation, my husband and I headed upstairs for my first outpatient oncology appointment. In our meeting with the oncologist, we all celebrated the end of radiation and the improvement in my back pain.

Once again, however, my husband and I were reminded that my treatment did not follow the conventional breast cancer drill. While most breast cancer patients undergo chemotherapy to prevent the cancer from spreading, my stage IV cancer diagnosis led my oncologist to combine the Tamoxifen I was taking with monthly treatment to my bones. She put me on Aredia, an osteo-porosis drug proven to help metastatic cancer patients stave off further spread of cancer within the bones. Although it's not che-motherapy, it is administered intravenously, just like chemother-apy. I was told that best-case scenario, I'd receive these monthly treatments for the next two years.

After meeting with the oncologist, my husband and I were ushered into the chemo room, a large open space with a couple dozen oversized chairs. Every chair was occupied. Most people in these chairs were bald; some had laptops, some had books. Some had family or friends sitting next to them. Others were alone. Despite the upbeat attitude of the nurses—who must have a seri-ously special gift to spend every work day in this room—the room reeked of grief.

I was scared, unsure of what this new treatment experience would be like. But the last month of hospital stays had also given me some perspective on my own condition: I had hair; I walked into the chemo room of my own accord; and most importantly, I was accompanied by a husband who held my hand, fetched me water, and smiled when he looked my way.

The room was packed with patients, so we were escorted to a semi-private sitting area, which I considered a small gift of grace. I had not been prepared for what I saw during this first visit to the chemo room and doubt I would have retained my composure had I been seated in the middle of the room.

After a couple failed attempts, the nurse finally found a suit-able vein and the IV began the *drip-drip-drip* into my veins. The nurse gave us an information card on Aredia, which we read repeatedly to help pass the time (new to the chemo room, we didn't know to bring the requisite bag of distractions—books, music, food—to occupy us). From the information card, we learned that the major side effect, especially the first time, is flu-like symptoms.

But we were heartened by terms like *rare* and *mild* scattered throughout the description. The explanation on the card was also supported by the oncologist's parting comments to us an hour before: "The drug shouldn't make you sick," she said reassuringly, accompanied by an encouraging nod of the head.

With the treatment complete, we headed downstairs in the hospital elevator for our third and final appointment of the day. My vertebroplasty was just three days away and I needed one final CT scan (a quick one this time, without the dye), which they would use to map out the surgery.

✓ A technician called my name, and as I followed him back to the scanner, he asked why I was there. When I told him I was scheduled for a vertebroplasty, he was visibly surprised, telling me that I looked forty years too young for such a procedure.

I gave him the thirty-second version of breast cancer's invasion of my back and the fracturing of my vertebrae. He stopped and stared at me, mouth open. Even though he recovered quickly and focused on getting me positioned for the scan, his response still made an impression, both in its humanity and its ability to unnerve me. I still haven't gotten used to being an anomaly to medical professionals.

After the scan the technician noted that my L2 vertebra was *pretty much obliterated*. Wanting to conclude on a positive note, he added that in his experience of working with patients with fractured backs, the vertebroplasty was a reliable pain-reducer and back-strengthener.

I appreciated his encouragement.

With all my hospital visits for the day completed, my husband and I returned home to celebrate the end of radiation with our girls.

The next morning I awoke to vicious flu-like symptoms that kept me in bed for two days, followed by a day of throwing up. With the vertebroplasty less than twenty-four hours away, my husband and I worried I wouldn't have the strength to go through with the procedure.

Monday morning, Martin Luther King Jr. Day, we called the spine surgeon, informing him of my lousy weekend. We asked whether or not we should go through with the procedure. He left the decision up to us. Motivated by assurances of a straighter, stronger back and further reduced pain, we decided to go ahead with the vertebroplasty.

The day at the hospital began in the spine surgeon's office, peering once again at MRI images of my L2 and L4 vertebrae. The surgeon informed us that he had recommended that the Intervention Radiologist (the doctor who would perform the vertebroplasty) inject the cement mixture only into the L2, the vertebra wholly destroyed by the cancer. The L4 was only partially destroyed, and the surgeon worried that the angle was less-than-optimal for getting the cement into the needed area. Prepped with this information, we headed downstairs for the procedure.

The Intervention Radiologist met with us before the procedure, confirming that the cement mixture would be injected into the L2 alone. The procedure itself took an hour, and I was "awake"—although once again I didn't remember much of the conversations the doctor later reported to me—so they could check in with me on pain and pressure.

My husband met me in the recovery room with a plush bathrobe in his arms, a gift from a former co-worker of his who had hand-delivered it to the hospital during the procedure. My husband draped the robe over my shoulders while the nurses tried to stabilize my pain. At first I asked for morphine rather than the Vicodin they were prepared to give me (Vicodin during the day continued to make me nauseous, and I was weary of the feeling); but three separate doses of morphine later my pain was still on the rise. I finally resorted to the Vicodin to diminish the pain. We returned home in time to get me into bed.

Morning came, and my husband and daughters all left the house to go live their lives.

Meanwhile the pain persisted at a staggering pitch. My spirits sank to the end of my toes. Rather than improving the level of pain, this procedure was inducing the opposite effect.

It also happened to be Inauguration Day, January 2009, and I anticipated that watching Barack Obama take the oath as our new president would be the day's one bright spot.

Mid-morning a friend called to ask how I was doing. She quickly surmised that things were not going well and offered to come over and keep me company. I was in need of company, but I had to be honest with my McCain-voting friend: I planned to watch Obama's inauguration and I wanted to be happy about it.

I heard the hesitation in her voice; certainly my plan for the day was not how my friend would choose to spend this frigid January day. But she came anyway, sitting next to me in front of the television, keeping my beverage glass cold, my compresses warm, my spirit steady, and her political opinions to a minimum.

High levels of pain accompanied me for the rest of the week. I felt awful. I cried at the drop of a hat.

My husband came home from work and, as I cried, looked searchingly into my eyes and asked, "Can you tell me why you're crying?"

I glared at him. Where had my bleary-eyed, emotional-train-wreck-of-a-husband gone? Just weeks before he had been a mess while I had been the resilient one. How could he go from a deluge of tears to wondering why *I* was crying?

Later that week, my husband and I talked about his emotional rebound. He told me he had recently had a realization: rather than spend his time grieving over a future without me while I was still around he had decided to focus on the present, on the time we had together, now.

While I knew I should be grateful for my husband's new grip on life, the truth was I didn't like it. My husband's spirits were rising just as mine were plummeting. If I was going to walk through the valley of the shadow of cancer, I wanted him there with me, not up ahead, in greener pastures, beside the still waters, with a restored soul.

Still, I tried to be happy for him. Certainly it was better for the girls to have a dad who had a grip. Undeniably it was better for my husband not to exhaust himself crying most of the day.

But I was scared to be in the pit of despair with no immediately discernable company.

About this same time I embarked on one of my first public outings since the diagnosis. My husband, my parents, and I headed to my older daughter's school for an award assembly. A couple weeks before, my daughter had come bursting through our front door, bouncing on her toes as she told me she had won a coveted school award. At a school where academics reign, this is the one award given for being an all-around good person. Our daughter had won this award in first grade, and now, six years later, was receiving it again.

Thrilled to be able to attend the ceremony, I sat, beaming, at the back of the cavernous school gym, buoyed by the hugs and enthusiastic greetings from teachers and parents alike.

We listened to classmate and teacher comments about the elementary award-winners of the good person award. When it finally came time for the junior high awards, the science teacher read off a list of characteristics about the winners: these students were kind, willing to help others, good friends, and had even *persevered through significant adversity.*

My smile faded.

I felt queasy.

Did my daughter just win an award because I have cancer?

Never mind the fact that my daughter's seven-year record at this school overflowed with honors; never mind that she *is* a good friend and willing to help others.

All I heard was that she got the award because I have cancer.

I felt sick, this time in my heart.

Could it be that cancer was now a defining aspect of my daughter's life as well as my own?

I hadn't yet allowed myself to think about how others would now see my daughter as a girl whose mother was really sick.

But my daughter did have a mother who was really sick. And she was being acknowledged for, among other things, persevering in the face of it.

At the time I couldn't digest the fact that my daughter's ability to maintain her composure—not to mention an A-plus average in all her classes—while our lives fell apart was indeed an award-worthy feat.

It wasn't until several weeks later, during a conference with our younger daughter's teacher—when we heard about her good days and bad days, and how the teachers strove to make school a safe place for her to be sad—did the effects of my cancer on our daughters really start to sink in.

I began to acknowledge that both my daughters were *persevering through adversity*, and I worked on being grateful they had teachers who cared enough to notice.

∽

February arrived and my first class was days away. Even though I was ecstatic to return to campus, I developed a mild panic about whether I'd be able to handle the demands of my spring course.

The day before class began, nausea kept me in bed. On the first day of class, my husband drove me to school, dropping me off just outside the door. In the minutes before class, colleagues gathered in and around my office, giving hugs and doling out offers of support.

My class meets right next to yours; if you need anything, just send a student over to get me.

Do you need anything carried to the classroom? I'm headed that way.

As I had experienced so many times in the past few months, my ability to stay standing—indeed, to stand at all—came from those who propped me up with their support, encouragement, prayers, and concern; and in these early days of spring semester, it was my colleagues who did the propping.

But by my own choice, I was the only teacher in the class-room. On that first day, I had planned to say something about my condition. Several of my students already knew, of course, but other students were new, not only to my classroom, but also to our university, transferring just in time for spring semester.

As the minutes ticked by, however, I couldn't muster the courage to say anything about cancer, back braces, or radiation. In fact, I focused most of my attention on making sure I wouldn't fall over during class.

I realized that day that my teaching style is a highly mobile one, and this pattern of constant movement made me increasingly unsteady on my feet as the class session went on. I knew I was weak, but I hadn't known how weak until I tried to stay on my feet for an hour.

Once class was over, my legs barely carried me back to my office. After collecting materials for the next class and answering a few emails, I called the colleague who had volunteered to take me home.

My colleague helped me out of the car and to my front door. I let myself into the house and climbed into bed.

Competing emotions followed me under the covers. On the one hand, I felt victorious: I had accomplished a significant feat to get back into the classroom, virtually my first "normal" act in the past two months. On the other hand, I was utterly at the mercy of my cancer-stricken body. I could barely teach or get dinner ready for my family or clean up or drive anywhere. While day one in the classroom was a victory, it was a small one.

As my February oncology appointment drew near, I was visited repeatedly by a vision. It went like this: I would enter the oncology waiting room, walk up to the appointment desk and hand over a stack of medical files. Then I would clear my throat and say, politely yet firmly: *I'm ready to give back my diagnosis. I've tried this cancer life on for size, and unfortunately, it doesn't fit my lifestyle. Thanks for your cooperation.* Surprised yet unprotesting, the receptionist would nod her head and take the file from me. I would turn around and march out of the oncology clinic and back into life as used to be.

On the day of the appointment, I couldn't get this scene out my head. I had had enough of cancer wreaking havoc on my life. I was sick of being sick.

I wanted no more chemo room visits where I had to sit next to other really sick people, hooked up to chemicals that would make each of us sicker before we might possibly get better. I wanted to teach without shaking. I wanted to be a mom of daughters who didn't need to persevere in the face of adversity. I wanted *out*, out of this world of cancer. I wanted to go back to when people told me how perfect my life was, to when I knew I was fortunate, to a time when life was good.

But there I was, a stage IV cancer patient, sitting in the oncology waiting room, without a single file to give back to the receptionist.

In the real-life version of the oncology visit, rather than insisting the receptionist take my files in return for my old life, I sat in the waiting room and cried. Tears streamed down my face for an hour straight as we waited to be called back for our appointment. My husband sat helplessly by my side, his hand on my leg, trying in vain to rub away the tears.

When the oncologist entered the exam room and saw my tear-stained face, she stopped, frowned, and said, "Oh dear. This isn't good. I think it might be time to see a counselor."

She went on to explain that the hospital had cancer counselors—psychologists who work exclusively with cancer patients—on staff and recommended I call and make an appointment with one of them.

Fabulous. Now I needed a special counselor to talk about my special cancer condition. The consequences of this new life never seemed to let up.

In the weeks that followed I experienced for the first time what I guessed were anxiety attacks. I couldn't sleep. I couldn't stop crying. I was losing my grip on this new life I wanted desperately to give away.

I would call the cancer counselor eventually, but not before I spent a few more weeks searching in vain for an exit route through this valley of the shadow of cancer.

seven

Embraced by the
Virtual Body of Christ

IN THE MIDST OF this foreign life in the land of cancer, teaching theology was the one remnant from my past that had been preserved more or less intact. Having resigned from virtually everything else that made my life rich with meaning, I treasured my three hours a week of class time where I could pretend that the rest of my life wasn't in ruins.

But even though I was teaching the same course I had taught many times before, the subject matter looked different from the first day of class on.

At the conclusion of the first class session, I asked students to take out a sheet of paper. "I'm going to read a few statements and I'd like you to write a brief response," I explained as I held on to the podium for extra support.

After the students pulled out some paper, I recited these words:

I believe in God, the Father Almighty, Maker of heaven and earth.

I believe in Jesus Christ, his only Son our Lord.

I believe in the Holy Spirit, the holy catholic church, the communion of saints, the forgiveness of sins.

Surveying the room full of puzzled faces, I moved to the instructions. "I want you to write about what comes to mind when you hear the words I just recited. Are you thinking: 'I've never heard these words before in my life'? or 'I believe these words, and say them every week'? Perhaps you've heard the words but don't understand what they mean. Or maybe you vaguely remember hearing these words when you were young and you used to believe them but now you're not so sure.

"Your responses won't be graded. This is just a way for me to get acquainted with you and for you to give me some information about your relationship with the theology we will be studying together this semester."

In typical undergraduate fashion, student responses ran the gamut from the enthusiastically devout to the seriously skeptical.

A number of students knew I had recited part of a creed; several even came up with its name: the Apostles' Creed. And most of the students who knew it was a creed wanted me to know they knew I had left certain parts out.

Among the students who understood their beliefs as mirroring the creed's confession, one wrote, *I believe most of what you said, except for that part about the Catholic Church. I wouldn't say I believe in the Catholic Church because I'm not Catholic.*

At the beginning of the next class session, I wrote *catholic* and *Catholic* on the blackboard. While the word *Catholic* does indeed refer to a specific institutional reality, we discussed that the word *catholic* actually means *universal*.

When Christians—whether Roman Catholic or not—recite the creed, I explained, they confess to believing in the church universal, a church that defies all boundaries and strictures commonly put on church. I concluded by suggesting that the church universal is a spiritual reality to which all Christians ultimately belong, even as they claim membership in specific churches.

This mini-lesson on the church catholic was intended to usher the class into the space where we would spend the rest of the semester: in the shifting sands between what the church and its people profess and how those professions of faith are embodied, revised, and even ignored in the lives of Christians now and in the past, here and far away.

As is the case most semesters, many of the students in this theology course didn't seem to grasp—or refused to buy into—the concept of the church universal. For lots of the students, it's an abstract, even off-putting idea. And for those students who had problems with specific churches—*that church is hypocritical; this one's too judgmental*—how much more problematic would it be to have a church with universal scope?

I have to admit that in life before cancer, I hadn't given the church universal much thought either. I could—and would—extol the virtues of participation in local communities of faith. I agree with theologians who say that the church is really being the church when it is present with those who suffer. As the daughter of a pastor, I have witnessed local churches time and again embody the hands and feet of Christ in their ministries to those in pain.

While my defense of the value of the local church used to come primarily from watching congregations bring Christ's love and care to *others* in need, I now have become a recipient of the church being the church in an intimately personal way.

In the weeks following my diagnosis, I slowly made my way back to Sunday morning worship at our church. Gentle hugs, warm hands grasping for ours, made us aware in tactile ways of God's embrace of us during this time of despair. When we came to the "Prayers of the People" during worship, my daughters' arms often found their way to my shoulders, while other friends seated nearby extended their arms, resting their hands on my back and arms. As my family and I heard my name offered up each week in prayer, we were reminded that our prayers were joined by the chorus of prayers surrounding us. To be accompanied by the church on this journey reassured me that we weren't walking alone. Their hands and feet became the hands and feet of Christ.

But through this cancer journey, I have also been awakened to a new—indeed, almost mystical—understanding of the church universal and the healing effects it has had on the lives of me and my family. The church universal is no longer an abstract, intangible concept glossed over during the reciting of the creed or mentioned briefly in class on the way to concepts that really matter.

Instead I have been surprised and humbled by the way in which the church universal has become a tangible agent of grace in my life, a gift that accompanied me through the valley of the shadow of cancer.

What has been most surprising to me is that the experience of the church universal has been mediated through what I'm calling *the virtual body of Christ*; that is, the body of Christ incarnated in, with, and through the power of Internet sites like CaringBridge.

Now let me be clear: I'm not trying to sound New Agey or to issue some feel-good platitude about how cancer has made me more appreciative of the value of community.

What I'm talking about is a new understanding of the church universal, a breathtakingly broad embodiment of Christ's hands and feet ministering amidst the sorrows and joys of life. I'm talking about Christ made present to me and my family through the connections made possible by a website.

This is not to say that before the Internet people were without the benefit of vast networks of prayers and support. But Internet connection has exponentially increased the speed and scope of such connections. And this more frequent communication—in my case, both with my updates and with the guestbook entries of encouragement—has been of immeasurable support to us since the diagnosis.

Not only have members of our own church been kept up-to-date through CaringBridge, but the website has made my story available to many other communities of faith, from the church where I grew up to the church my husband and I joined during graduate school in Nashville to my in-laws church in Duluth and to a friend's church outside Chicago.

Because of the CaringBridge journal and guestbook entries, toddlers in Portland knew my story and said my name in their nightly prayers; students and staff at a girls' school in Baltimore heard my story and included my name in Friday worship, even relatives in Sweden and Norway received regular updates via CaringBridge and held us regularly in prayer.

As readership of the CaringBridge site grew, prayer shawls from other churches were delivered to our home; we now have six of them, more than one for each member of the family. These shawls confirm for us again and again the mysterious support and power of the church universal.

This experience of the virtual body of Christ has also gifted me with a fresh appreciation of the necessarily ecumenical character of church catholicity. Prompted by my entries on the CaringBridge site, many of my friends from the Roman Catholic tradition—the church that holds most tightly to this notion of universality—have embodied Christ to me in stunning ways.

Since the news of my diagnosis spread via CaringBridge, I have had Mass dedicated to me in India, Sri Lanka, California, and the Twin Cities; I have received hundreds of cards from one California parish where Sunday School classes prayed for me weekly; and I have been given a medallion blessed and sent on to me by a priest friend. These traditions of dedicating, blessing, and honoring—traditions that make rare appearances in our Protestant expressions of church—have made their mark on my soul. To hold the "With God, all things are possible" medallion from my priest friend brings deep comfort.

But there is still more to say about the universal nature of the church. In the months since my diagnosis, I have had a growing conviction that this notion of the church universal extends even further, beyond the bounds of Christian communities to include those of other faiths and even those of no particular faith.

With this assertion I realize I'm wading into murky waters; after all, most Christians would say that talk of the church universal needs to involve the profession of Christ somewhere, someway.

But I have no intention of taking Christ out of Christianity and most definitely not out of church. If Christ remains at the center, however, suggesting that the church universal includes non-Christians could look like I'm claiming that friends outside Christianity are actually part of the church even if they don't want to be.

I don't have all the details worked out yet, but what I do know is this: my friends and colleagues of other faiths, and even those who claim no faith at all, have included me in their prayers, their rituals, their sacred practices. And I can find no other language in my theological lexicon that's up to the task of describing their ministry to me and my family.

What I *am* ready to do is begin rethinking my own beliefs in light of the boundary-breaking experiences of grace I have encountered since my diagnosis.

Take the grace bestowed upon me by one of my agnostic Jewish colleagues. Her gift to me began with the CaringBridge site; it includes Christ in a profound way; and it takes me beyond the bounds of the church universal conventionally understood.

Shortly after this Jewish colleague of mine returned from a study abroad trip to Israel with a group of our students, she sent me an email message. The message began with a disclaimer about how she has never been a very religious person. From her childhood in Israel to her adult life here in the U.S., she has attended synagogue but often felt on the outside of explicitly religious practices like prayer.

I was intrigued by the story of my colleague's uneasy relationship with religion but unsure as to why she was taking the time to share the story with me. Even though she and I had worked together for over a dozen years, we had had few in-depth conversations and none of them had been about religion.

I read on.

My colleague wrote next about my postings on CaringBridge and about how my journey with cancer—and along with it, my struggles with my own faith—had become a source of inspiration to her. Spurred on by my story, she had even gone out on a limb and attempted to pray herself.

I was startled to learn that the public narration of my journey with cancer—a task I found difficult, especially when it came to talking about faith—had become an impetus for the deepening of this colleague's own spiritual journey.

But that wasn't all there was to the message.

All of the information about my colleague's struggles with religion and the inspiration she drew from reading my journals was mere backdrop for what she was about to tell me about her trip to Israel.

She went on to describe the group's day at the Western Wall in Jerusalem. She told me that she and another colleague had placed prayers for me into the cracks in the wall. She wrote about how moved she was to see several of our students add their prayers for me to the wall as well.

To learn that prayers for me had even made it to the Western Wall was profoundly moving. We Christians trace our spiritual inheritance back to the Jews who built that very wall. Knowing Jesus prayed and studied above that wall and that prayers for me remain in the city of Jerusalem—a holy city to both Jews and Christians (and Muslims, too)—further supported my widening view of the church universal.

But my colleague had not yet come to her main point.

She wrote about how in their travels throughout Israel the group had visited many churches in addition to synagogues and mosques. And much to my surprise and even to her own, the churches they visited became places where she tried out her newly acquired practice of prayer.

In each church her group visited, my colleague told me, she would sit down, bow her head, and ask Jesus for a favor: that he might consider healing her friend with cancer.

Her message to me ended with this: *I hope I didn't offend Jesus—after all, I'm a Jew and I don't even pray regularly—and there I was, asking Jesus for a favor. I think he'll be o.k. with that, won't he?*

Stunned, I reread the message, making sure I hadn't inadvertently rearranged the words.

I hadn't. My agnostic Jewish colleague had indeed written to tell me that she had prayed to Jesus and asked him for a favor. *For me.*

Words still elude me when I try to describe what this act of prayer has meant to me. And I'm convinced it has to fit somewhere inside a theology of the church universal. But just where or how it fits I'm not so sure.

When I told another Jewish friend of mine about my colleague's request of Jesus, she looked at me incredulously and declared, "But she doesn't even know Jesus!"

That may be. At the same time, it seems that my Jewish colleague entered into some kind of relationship—however tentative or uneasy—with this Jewish man Christians call Healer and Savior.

I realize it's tricky and complicated, but for this particular Christian there's no other way to say it: knowing Jesus was asked a favor for me by a Jewish colleague bears saving love, saving presence, and saving hope to me in a time of deep brokenness, struggle, and despair. This beautiful act has to be bound up somehow, someway, to God's universal community of saints; it's too much like Christ for it to be any other way.

When it comes to the church universal, then, my understanding has been broken open to a new beyond—beyond what we Christians are able to imagine, beyond tidy categories of what counts as religious and what doesn't.

Since the diagnosis, I've received a sage blessing from a Native American colleague, been prayed for in the synagogues of friends and colleagues, had Buddhist meditation sessions dedicated to me; and Jesus has even been asked a favor by a Jewish friend who took a gamble on my behalf.

I don't know what else to call it but grace. And these gifts of grace from the virtual body of Christ enabled me to keep walking through the valley of the shadow of cancer, even through the darkest days of a Minnesota winter.

eight

Getting to Easter

As a Minnesotan, I've always hated February. Everyone expects it to be cold in January; then February rolls around and in Minnesota, winter shows no signs of letting up. I lived in Nashville during graduate school and was shocked to discover that spring started to stir in February. In Minnesota in February, spring is still years away.

On top of the arctic weather, February also ushers in the church season of Lent, which as a theologian I strongly approve of. Theoretically. It is important to pare down, do without, take stock of our sin, and reflect on the suffering of Jesus. But practically speaking, it's the downer season of the church year. I'm Lutheran and Lutherans are big on sin, but when Lent comes in the middle of a Minnesota February, I dream of practicing another faith in another state.

Ash Wednesday arrived and I couldn't muster up the courage to go to church. The thought of approaching the altar so that one of our pastors could make the sign of the cross on my forehead and say, "You are dust and to dust you shall return," was more than I could handle this particular February. Two of my vertebrae had already turned to ashes and I feared the rest of me wasn't far behind. I needed no additional reminder that death was near.

So our nine-year-old—grateful for a chance to skip the ash-signing this year—offered to stay with me while my husband and older daughter went to church. She and I snuggled up together on the couch and read a book that wasn't about ashes, Lent, or February.

Soon after Lent began, I visited the cancer counselor. A long-time friend picked me up and drove me to the hospital for the appointment. A couple minutes after we were seated in the waiting room, the counselor arrived, shook my hand and the hand of my friend and introduced herself. As she and I walked back to her office, the counselor turned to me and said, "I can tell your friend loves you fiercely."

Her words knocked me off balance and I struggled to keep up with her as we approached her office. *It's true*, I thought, *my friend does love me fiercely. I'm loved fiercely by so many in my life right now, and I'm more miserable than I've ever been in my forty-two years.*

I also knew I had no idea how to move beyond the awful place I was in.

The counselor asked me to tell my story, which required lots of tears. She understood right away the gravity of my situation and told me that she could help me deal with the pragmatics of life with stage IV cancer. Even more immediate than questions about the future, the counselor explained, was whether I'd have a bowel movement today or whether I'd sleep tonight (I perked up: these were exactly my most pressing concerns).

I told her of my failed attempts at sleep, and she leaned forward and insisted, "When you have stage IV cancer, you should be sleeping *by any means necessary*. Your body needs all the energy it can muster to fight this, and if you're not sleeping, your body can't heal."

I have a basic aversion to medication (giving birth to my first child without anesthetics), a position at serious cross-purposes with my new life as a cancer patient. But I listened and told her I would consider the recommendation.

The counselor also asked how my relationships were faring. I talked of the enormous support I had received from all corners of my life. I also admitted to some challenging moments with family and friends. I recounted the conversation my husband and I had had during my second hospital stay, telling her how he hadn't appreciated my suggestion he find someone else after I die.

The counselor nodded her head knowingly and said, "Your response is understandable, but your timing was all wrong." Rather than initiating such painful conversations in the present, the counselor recommended purchasing a black box and some lovely stationery so I could write letters to my husband for him to read after my death.

The counselor encouraged me to write letters to my daughters as well. "One letter can be titled, 'On Your Graduation Day,'" she explained, "and another, 'On Your Wedding Day.' You can start these letters with 'I wish I were here with you today. Know that if I were, these are some of the things I would say . . .'"

The black-box-filled-with-letters suggestion caught me off guard. I was quite sure this cancer counselor knew more about stage IV cancer than I did, and the fact that she was instructing me to spend my time *now*—two months after my diagnosis, just when my body was beginning to show initial signs of healing— writing letters to my family about life without me was sobering. I had many things to say to my husband and my daughters about events in the future but I still held out hope that I might be able to say them *in person*. Striving to be a good patient, I considered this suggestion as well: perhaps it was time for me to start writing letters to leave behind.

As we wrapped up our conversation, the counselor told me she suspected I had "trauma-induced depression" (shocking) and proposed I see her again in a few weeks. As we said our good-byes the counselor offered one last piece of advice: "And don't worry about whether or not these visits will be covered by insurance," she said in a reassuring tone. "With stage IV cancer, that's all the justification for counseling you need."

Walking to the car, my friend asked me how the session had gone.

I chose my words carefully. "It was good to do," I said slowly. "I think she wants to help me figure out how to live while preparing to die."

The problem was I didn't see my death as imminent as she apparently did. I also wasn't sure this was the right time to focus on words from the grave to my husband and daughters. But I was no expert at having stage IV cancer and the counselor spends her days advising people like me. After a brief discussion of the visit with my friend, I changed the subject, setting aside the counselor's suggestions for later.

That night I told my husband about the counseling session. He listened intently to my report, appreciating the advice about sleep medication. But when I got to the part about the black box and writing notes to him on pretty stationery about my hopes for his life post-me, he looked at me incredulously and exclaimed, "*No way!* Even though I didn't *like* hearing that you hope I find someone else after you die, I still want you to tell me what you're thinking. I don't want to find some little black box after you're gone that holds your thoughts on the future," he scoffed. "I want us to have all those conversations now, before you go."

Disgusted with the counselor's advice, my husband urged us to take a different approach to handling the hard topics cancer had introduced into our lives.

My husband's reaction caught me off guard as well, but his rant against the box full of letters brought some relief. Perhaps I will write letters for my family to read after I die, but my husband gave me permission to take the task off the immediate "to do" list.

As I continued to lay awake for hours each night, I considered the counselor's advice about sleep medication. I finally called the oncologist and got a prescription for Ambien. I wrote about this development on my CaringBridge site and received numerous messages of support from friends and colleagues who cited their own use of sleep medication and on which drugs worked best.

The first night on Ambien, I slept a staggering seven hours straight. I felt like a new person. *Why hadn't I done this weeks ago?* I wondered. Ambien became my new best friend.

Several days later, I received an email from a colleague following my story on CaringBridge. She shared with me her troubles with Ambien, writing about night terrors she believed were brought on by Ambien and about the long and painful process of going off this drug.

Just that morning, I had experienced the most severe attack of anxiety since the diagnosis. I wondered if my spike in anxiety could be related to the Ambien. That night I set the Ambien aside and returned to over-the-counter medication.

I didn't sleep well but felt much calmer the next day. I decided that sleeping better was not worth the price of higher anxiety. I called the oncologist and told her about the side effects of Ambien. She moved me on to Trazadone, another sleep medication. I wrote more about my struggle with sleep on CaringBridge. Many more readers wrote in, some testifying to Trazadone's efficacy, others voting for alternative medications.

The responses in the guestbook were reassuring: I certainly wasn't the only one with sleep problems. In fact, "the whole world seems to be on sleep meds," my husband observed after making it through all the messages posted on my site that week.

Trazadone helped me sleep during the night but left me groggy and listless in the morning. A week later, I added the bottle of Trazadone to my growing closet pharmacy and returned to over-the-counter sleep options along with some essential oils sent by a mother of one my daughter's friends. I would wait until the next oncology appointment to talk about other prescriptive options.

My difficulty sleeping did nothing to help my low opinion of February. During a typical winter, I work against my mid-winter blues by heading outdoors and enjoying the cold and snow. While my husband spends most of his leisure wintertime indoors watching college basketball and dreaming of golf, I spend my winters making frequent trips with the girls to the sledding hill, ice rink, and ski slope. But here it was the middle of February and the only safe place for me was in a climate-controlled environment free of ice.

This is why walking indoors became increasingly important to my daily routine. I walked with my husband, my parents, my daughters, my in-laws, friends and colleagues.

One friend in particular stood at the center of this activity. She and I had met years earlier, when our children attended the same preschool. She is also a professor and had started a year-long sabbatical from teaching in the fall. As the leaves turned colors, we renewed our friendship during walks together along the Mississippi River. We caught up on each other's lives, swapping experiences about teaching college students and raising fourth-grade girls.

From the day of my diagnosis onward, however, I don't know whether she or I was more grateful for her sabbatical. She made herself available for weekly—and sometimes twice weekly—walks. She would pick me up, drive to the mall, and literally accompany me each step along paths of sorrow, grief, anger, pain and hope.

I remember one ride to the mall when I started to wail and couldn't stop. I was completely undone. My friend placed her hand on my knee and assured me she would continue to be there for me. Through the worst of the winter my friend kept walking with me, no matter where the walk led.

The regularity of our walks also allowed me to work through my evolving perspective on my new life. It took me a while to catch on, but eventually I realized that my friend would listen to me talk about the challenges coming my way—from my reaction to the osteoporosis drug to my uncertainty about whether or not I should get a mastectomy—and before our next walk, she would research these issues and show up for our next walk with volumes of new information.

A couple months into the new year, it dawned on me that during every walk, my friend would say something like, "that's in line with what I've read" or "that's different from the research I've seen on that issue." In addition to being a faithful friend and walking partner, my friend was also serving as an ultra-competent researcher of my condition. Her research educated me on a range of issues related to my condition, which helped enormously as I processed the next steps in this cancer journey.

While cancer dominated our discussions, my friend and I occasionally took time for other topics, too. During one walk around the mall, this friend told me about a religion test her daughter had taken at the Catholic school she attended. They had been studying saints and the final question on the test asked students to name a saint. In the answer blank, my friend's daughter had written the words, "My Mother." The test was returned with "My Mother" marked wrong in red ink.

Granted my friend does not fit the technical definition of a saint—she hasn't taken vows of poverty, chastity, or obedience; she hasn't performed a miracle recognized by the church. To be honest, she's not even Catholic, reticent to claim any religious affiliation at all. Furthermore, I know teaching religion can be tricky; there are facts about religion and there's truth beyond the facts, and sometimes it's hard to do justice to both.

At the same time, in my mind this fourth-grade teacher passed up a valuable learning opportunity with this group of students. In teaching the facts of sainthood, I imagine the teacher talked of saints as those whose extravagant love, service, healing, and sacrifice was officially recognized by the church. But a truth-beyond-the-facts presented itself in the "My Mother" answer, for what could be more wonderful than a child's belief that her parent embodies such saintly qualities? I for one am with my friend's daughter: her mother's a saint.

❦

Even with my daily walks with my saintly friend and other loved ones, I continued to be beaten down by the cancer-winter-Lent triple threat.

But over President's Day weekend, my husband, daughters, and I headed south, to Tucson, Arizona, where my aunt and uncle had offered their condominium for our use. Our plane landed after midnight and we fell into bed as soon as we had unlocked the front door. When morning arrived, the four of us migrated to the living room and opened the floor-to-ceiling shades covering the windows. What appeared took our breath away: a panoramic view of the Santa Catalina Mountains.

After marveling at the scenery, we headed for the kitchen where we found a note from my uncle detailing where to hike, what to eat, and how to drive the Jeep. We took his recommendation and brought our breakfast out onto the backyard patio overlooking the mountains. It wasn't balmy—the temperature was in the 50s—but we were outside, in the sunshine, without winter jackets. It was going to be a fabulous weekend.

Later that morning we drove to Sabino Canyon, a popular hiking spot in the area. We purchased passes for the tram and rode deep into the canyon. We got off at the last stop, eager to try a little hiking. Our family vacations almost always involve mountains and hiking, but we all knew that my hiking abilities were severely limited. Nevertheless, we reveled in being outside. We walked along the Telephone Line Trail, stopping frequently to admire the scenery.

In the early afternoon, we found a rock suitable for sitting and ate lunch. Revived by the food, we continued on and before we knew it we had hiked a good two miles of the canyon. It was exhilarating, and we were all amazed I was still standing. We rested alongside a pool of water. The girls shed their shoes and waded in.

Sitting on the rock, breathing in the warm air, watching my daughters smile into the sun, I felt a small surge of hope; maybe we could live again in a world not dominated by cancer.

The rest of the weekend was more of the same: lounging around the condo in the morning, exploring the desert by day and enjoying evenings indoors, reading, playing games, watching movies. Heading to the airport Monday afternoon we all felt rejuvenated by our time in the sun, grateful for the respite from icy Minnesota and the cancer-filled life that awaited our return.

❧

Back in the Twin Cities, the girls and I returned to school and my husband, to work. The week quickly arrived at Thursday, the day when two longtime friends from graduate school were flying in to see me.

In January my friends had written to tell me that they planned to come and spend a weekend with me. Learning of their plans brought more tears to my eyes. We had met in seminary; both of them had prepared for the ministry while I pursued the teaching route. In the almost-two decades since our seminary days, there were four of us women who had stayed in touch, recently gathering our families for New Years on the Delaware shore in celebration of our fortieth birthdays.

At one point during our Delaware reunion weekend the four of us found ourselves walking along the beach, deep in the type of conversation we used to have time for in graduate school. One friend asked how our lives now compared with our vision for our lives back when we first met.

That the joys of the past fifteen years had been accompanied by sorrow was central to the stories told by each of my three friends. From the loss of pre-term babies to struggles with postpartum depression to the pain of losing a parent, my friends' lives were punctuated by the still-present grief of these events.

Toward the end of our walk one of my friends turned to me and said, "Your life seems to have gone just like you envisioned it would, hasn't it?"

Even though I felt a bit convicted by her question, there was no accusation in my friend's voice. Her observation was simply an affirmation of the good life I was living.

Knowing how terribly my life had recently veered off course, these friends were on their way to spend the weekend with me.

I drove to the airport to pick up my friends, one of my first attempts at driving since the diagnosis. We drove from the airport to dinner at a neighborhood restaurant, my first restaurant dining experience in months. The weekend of talking, crying, eating, and laughing with my longtime minister friends was like a long exhale after months of inhaling. Together they offered a potent balance of counsel, friendship, ministerial insight, and comic relief. I leaned into their embrace, and they held me, along with the grief and the grace that had come to bracket my life.

The week that began with inhaling the warm desert air with my family ended with exhaling some of the grief over my new life in the presence of old friends. I started to glimpse the possibility that Easter might actually be on its way.

∾

What had initially been a frightening prospect—teaching my theology class— became integral to my slow steps toward healing. During the first month of class, teaching was the only activity that got me out of bed and dressed for the day. Outside the classroom, my colleagues lovingly and graciously encouraged me. Inside the classroom I was blessed with one of the most mature, inquisitive, and good-natured group of students I'd had in a long time. Their enthusiastic engagement with me and with the theology we studied reassured me that cancer had not yet claimed all of my life.

In a typical semester, my personal life makes regular appearances in the classroom. This is not just because I like to talk about myself; rather, getting personal is actually part of our religion department's pedagogical approach. One of the many things I love about our department is that all of us identify as scholar-practitioners; that is, we don't just teach religion, we also practice it. In the dual role of scholar and practitioner we seek to model for our students how the study of religion can positively impact a life of faith and vice versa.

But as a department where our faculty represent multiple faith traditions (Jewish, Buddhist, and Christian) we are also clear that acknowledging our experiences as practitioners of faith is not for purposes of proselytizing, nor is it to coerce our students into thinking—or practicing—like we do. Instead, illustrations from our lives as religious practitioners serve the larger goal of understanding religious traditions from the inside out, through the lens of persons committed to its practice.

This semester, however, I had been reticent about getting personal. My life was overrun by cancer—except, that is, in the classroom. Theology class had become the only place where cancer seemingly didn't reach, and I wasn't eager to disturb the classroom's "cancer-free" environment.

But as we approached the topic of theodicy—theories about God's relationship to sin and suffering—I sensed cancer would soon make an appearance. Our treatment of theodicy began with a review of the most common explanations of God's relationship to suffering. We looked first at the "hard times make you strong" response to suffering. In this view God sends trials and suffering our way to build character and make us stronger. As a class we discussed why people embrace this response. Several students pointed to the need to know there's a reason for the suffering; others suggested that if God is all-powerful and involved in our lives then suffering and God have to be linked.

After affirming these views as representative of many people's faith, I paused. "But do *you* buy this view?" I asked them. Some nodded, familiar with this view of God and the worldview that supports it. Others looked skeptical.

"Certainly most of us can look back on difficult times in our lives and see that we have become stronger because of them. Sometimes challenges are good and help us grow," I encouraged them.

"But do the hard times always lead to growth?"

The room fell silent.

"Is God responsible for sending people suffering that robs them of their dignity? For the pain that strips them clean?"

It was time.

"As some of you know," I continued, "I've been dealing with cancer over the past few months"—I had opened the door; now I needed to walk through it—"and some people have taken this approach with me, suggesting God has given me cancer to make me a stronger person.

"Personally, I don't buy it. Cancer sucks, and I have a hard time believing in a God who sends people cancer or other terminal illness in order to teach them a lesson. This view simply does not acknowledge the full scope of suffering that pervades many of our lives."

During this final sentence, my voice became a bit shaky, and I knew I was fast approaching my limit of personal disclosure for the day. So I did what teachers do when they reach an impasse: I asked another question.

"Why might those who suffer find this view of God and suffering inadequate?"

The students knew we were getting somewhere. They jumped in, suggesting that while God might be all powerful, Scripture also emphasizes God's love, and a God whose love knows no bounds seems at serious odds with a God who wills cancer, AIDS, earthquakes, and other sources of death and destruction on us.

Toward the end of class, we considered the theological response to suffering proposed by our text. Our author called for a more thorough-goingly biblical response to God and suffering than is offered by the theories we had reviewed. Instead, he proposes a portrait of God that focuses on God's journey to

the depths of human suffering, pain, and alienation in the death
of Jesus.

Standing within the biblical story, he says, Christians are
called to look at God's relationship to suffering through the lens
of Jesus' life, where God takes suffering into God's very being but
refuses to let death have the last word. God brings new life out of
the tragic death of Jesus, not to teach us a lesson about suffering,
not as some guarantee that suffering can be avoided. In the life,
death, and resurrection of Jesus, God takes on human sin and suffering, ultimately overcoming them through the gift of new life.

Our theologian ends his chapter on God and suffering with
the insistence that in the face of real, deep experiences of suffering, theories are simply not enough. Faith involves a relationship with a God who suffers with us and refuses to leave it—or
us—unredeemed.

As class came to a close, I could tell some of my students
were on board with our theologian's view. Other students didn't
buy it. For the skeptics, claiming allegiance to a God who ultimately overcomes suffering and death was not enough either.

One student suggested that Christian faith is ultimately a
kind of wager. In faith Christians wager that God accompanies us
in our suffering and that through Christ, God promises that sin,
death, and destruction will not triumph in the end. For some of
my students, such a wager was too big a gamble. For others, it's an
outrageous claim lacking sufficient evidence.

But for still others, they—like me—were working to stake
their lives on it.

As I headed back to my office after class I realized I had
started to embrace the season of Lent, along with a growing
awareness that embracing Lent meant embracing not just sin, suffering, and death, but the assurance that Easter has the final word.

∾

My self-divulging in class was possible not only because I had developed a rapport with the students but also because outside of class, I was beginning to be able to talk about faith in light of having cancer.

For the first two months after the diagnosis I was speechless before God. The best I could do in the faith department was wear one of my prayer shawls and pray along with prayers of others.

But with help from my mother I used words of the psalmist to get me back on speaking terms with God.

Even though I didn't talk much about the spiritual side of my struggle, my mom could tell what was going on. She was over at our house almost daily and as someone who had walked a similar path with cancer she knew well that the physical challenges were only half the battle.

During Lent, my mom, a recent entrant into the world of email communication, sent regular messages to me recounting how sustained prayer and meditation had helped her through the worst days of her own cancer treatments. She shared with me how she had memorized psalms, reciting them every day in a slow, meditative way. She typed out the psalms for me word-for-word, explaining where she sat, how she breathed, and what she imagined as she prayed.

As cancer threatened to take her health and even her life, my mom journeyed deeper into relationship with Jesus, whom she envisioned as overcoming the cancer. And now she was sharing her journey into deeper faith with me.

My mom's messages provided me with words to begin speaking with God again. I began tentatively, realizing that I wasn't sure what trusting God meant in a life with cancer. As a theologian, I have spent much time with the question of God's relationship to suffering, knowing all along that I had precious little actual experience from which to draw. In truth, for years I feared that my relative inexperience with suffering meant that when it finally came—as it inevitably does—suffering would come so ferociously into my life it would knock me down.

And here I was, knocked down by a diagnosis of stage IV cancer.

I haven't spent much time asking "Why me?" for I don't believe God caused my cancer. At the same time, as I began to talk again to God I was acutely aware of the feeling of God's absence. I have also read much theological reflection on the absence of God. But living it is not the same as reading about it. What does it mean to trust in a God who seems to be non-responsive?

I ache, and God is silent. What do I do now?

I remember hearing at some youth event back in high school that "if God seems far away, you're the one who's moved." That may be an effective comment in some situations, but I knew that since the diagnosis, I hadn't moved of my own accord. Cancer had moved me to a place where conversations with God were at an impasse.

At the same time I was aware of being held up over and over again by what I consider to be the Spirit working in and through doctors, technicians, family, friends, neighbors. Being held up gave me reason to thank God. But it was time to say more than "thanks."

This is where the psalms came in. While many would argue that the words of the twenty-third psalm have become ubiquitous and thus cliché, I was nevertheless drawn into the imagery and the psalm's ability to account for the depths—*even though I walk through the valley of the shadow of death*—as well as for the comfort sought by those who suffer. The psalmist's talk of God's preparation of a table for us in the presence of our enemies captured my struggle to embrace the daily gifts of grace spread out before me in the presence of cancer. *Surely goodness and mercy shall follow me all the days of my life* challenged me daily, as my life seemed devoid of much of its former goodness and mercy.

Nevertheless, I recited the entire psalm daily, trying to rest in the promise of dwelling *in the house of the Lord forever.*

Borrowing words from the psalms for daily meditation and prayer slowly began to renew my spirit. I still didn't fully understand what trusting God in the midst of stage IV cancer meant but I had embarked on the path of finding out.

As my spirit slowly improved so did my physical mobility and stamina. I finally weaned myself off prescriptive pain meds. I talked again with the spine surgeon and he encouraged me to take off the back brace a few hours a day, gradually extending my time without it.

I started with baby steps, getting out of bed and eating breakfast brace-less, then putting it on when I got dressed. I took the brace off when I sat on the couch and graded papers. I took it off at night when I watched a little television. Then one morning a friend picked me up for a walk at the mall. I climbed in her van, realizing minutes later I was without my brace. "Oh, no!" I exclaimed. Then it occurred to me that if I hadn't thought about the brace until then perhaps I could take a few laps around the mall without it.

Thus began the first day of my life without the brace. By evening I needed some ibuprofen, but other than the dull, mild pain, my back felt surprisingly steady without its extra support.

ᔕ

March arrived, and along with it, my third oncology appointment. In February I had skipped the scheduled osteoporosis treatment; I didn't think I could bear more negative side effects. But with strong encouragement from my husband and others I decided to try again, this time with a different osteoporosis drug, Zometa, hoping the side effects would be less severe.

The appointment began with a blood test that checked the cancer markers in my blood for the first time since the day of the diagnosis. My husband and I learned that people who are cancer free should have a cancer marker of zero, a long way from the 256-marker found in my blood at my diagnosis in December.

We were not told explicitly how bad 256 was, but we learned that remission is anything under thirty-eight. Any way you count it, my markers had been high in the danger zone.

The day after my appointment the nurse called with the results: my cancer markers had dropped significantly, from 256 to ninety-six. The nurse told me the decreasing markers indicated that my body was responding well to the treatments I was receiving. We exhaled again.

But not completely. I had awakened once again to flu-like symptoms. My friend from the university was supposed to pick me up and go walking with me at the mall; instead she came to the house. She let herself in and came up to my bedroom where she found me in bed, tears flowing. My friend has a gift for righteous anger and let some of it fly when she saw me confined again to bed.

"*That stupid medication.* It's not supposed to do this! You were supposed to feel much better this time. This is *so stupid.*"

Her anger helped me regain my composure. After weeks of feeling stronger every day, I was unnerved at how quickly I was knocked out again. Every time I started thinking I was gaining on cancer, it seemed to reassert itself to make sure I knew who was calling the shots.

But the nausea and aching abated much more quickly this time, which allowed my family and me to focus on the declining cancer markers. The news had a positive psychological effect on all of us. Maybe my stage IV cancer didn't mean imminent death. Maybe I could hold off writing those letters for the black box a while longer.

As far as sleep medication was concerned, the third time was a charm. The oncologist gave me a prescription for Lunesta, which allowed me to sleep well and awake with little-to-no grogginess. Sleeping six or more hours a night allowed March to look significantly different than February.

Holy week arrived. My older daughter, now part of our church youth group, played the role of Mary Magdalene in a Good Friday passion play at church. My parents, husband, younger daughter, and I all attended the performance, standing in the midst of the scenes as the story moved from the marketplace to the upper room, to the garden, and finally, to Golgatha, the place where Jesus was killed. Our daughter fully embodied the part of Mary, loyal to Jesus until the end, full of grief at his death.

As I watched my daughter and the rest of the seventh and eighth graders reenact the drama I was reminded of a Good Friday service we attended with her when she was barely three years old. The pastor's sermon began with the words, "Good Friday was not a good day for Jesus." In the dramatic pause that followed, our almost-three-year-old spoke clearly and thoughtfully into the silence.

"Why wasn't it a good day for Jesus?"

In the midst of the polite chuckles that followed, I caught a glimpse of the deeply spiritual person she would become. Her question was earnest; she wanted a serious answer. Now here she was, years later, showing us all how bad Good Friday really was for those who loved Jesus.

With the help of our daughter's performance and a passionate portrayal of Jesus (by a girl, no less), we left church keenly aware of the lack of resolution in Good Friday. For the time being, sin, suffering, despair, and death have the upper hand. Taken on its own, there's no good news on Good Friday.

But for Christians, Good Friday's darkness and despair is ultimately overcome—but not forgotten—by Easter.

We awoke Easter morning to a gorgeous spring day, a day I had doubted would ever arrive. But here it was. Easter.

My younger daughter had chosen Easter Sunday to celebrate her First Communion. In the Lutheran tradition we talk about Christ being really present in the bread and wine of communion. And despite my daughter's eagerness to complete this rite of passage in her spiritual life, she waited until Easter Sunday—the last possible date—to experience this presence at a new and deeper level.

I teared up as we walked forward for our Easter communion. Here my daughter would receive Christ's broken body. She would ask for forgiveness for the brokenness in her life.

But she had decided that her first communion with Christ's body and blood would come on Easter morn, amidst proclamations that brokenness is not the end of the story. She chose a day full of Alleluias to the risen Christ, the one who offers new life, the one who's really present with her on this day and always.

The rest of Easter was rich with family—my parents worshiping with us and my husband's parents and sister's family spending Easter dinner at our house (our hosting responsibilities included setting the table and providing beverages—my husband's family did the rest) and with friends to whom we delivered Easter bouquets as small signs of our appreciation of their love and support.

As my husband and I climbed into bed at the end of the day, I was able to give him a genuine smile for the first time in months. We still didn't know what our future of living with stage IV cancer looked like. But this we did know: for this year, February was over. And so was Lent.

He smiled back. Easter had finally arrived.

nine

Having Cancer, Talking Cancer

IN ONE CANCER MEMOIR I read, the author writes about the scene in the exam room after she learns she has breast cancer. She looks at the doctor through her tears and whispers, "I'm sorry. I just don't know how to have cancer." The doctor puts his hand on her shoulder and says, "None of us knows how to have cancer."

None of us knows how to have cancer.

It's a humble and humbling claim, one I seek comfort in, both in terms of my own bewilderment over how to cope with cancer in my own life and in the lives of others, as well as the challenge of how to deal with those who mean well but offer little comfort at all.

I don't want to say it's all relative when it comes to cancer, but those of us with cancer experience and cope with the disease and its effects in wildly different ways. Some passionately protect their privacy; others are exceedingly public with the details. Some head to work every day during treatment; others' lives come to a halt. But something we all share is this: the havoc that cancer creates in our lives and in the lives of those who love—or simply interact with—us.

How, then, do you have cancer? And how do you talk about it?

On good days, when someone makes a comment I disagree with or says something insensitive or just plain wrong, I remind myself that none of us knows how to have cancer.

On good days, I realize a person who makes an inappropriate comment overcame the temptation to say nothing at all, which (theoretically) I appreciate. Rather than ignoring my cancer, this person—however awkwardly—is acknowledging cancer's invasion into my life.

On good days, I attempt to be gracious, even when the comments sting. I'm a professor; I adopt an educative role, explaining why their point of view differs from my own.

The problem is not all days are good days.

In fact, many days with cancer are bad days. On those days, I'm not so magnanimous in my response. Rather than greeting awkward attempts at consolation with gravitas, I get offended, angry, hurt.

On bad days, my retorts to off-the-mark comments often offend in return. Close friends and family tell me I have no reason to feel badly about my sharp replies. That it's not my job to take care of others and their misguided assumptions.

But it's not that easy: none of us knows how to have cancer.

I talked with the cancer counselor about some of the unwelcome comments I have heard, and she shared with me her list of the top ten stupid things people say about cancer. She encouraged me to call people out, even when such an approach goes against the grain of "Minnesota nice" (a nomenclature that, depending on your perspective, refers to Minnesotans' understated kindness or to a passive aggressive tendency that masquerades as *nice* on the surface). Clearly not from Minnesota herself, the counselor wondered whether "F--k you!" could become part of my repertoire.

I laughed, shaking my head from side to side, recalling how a faculty colleague of mine had peppered his guest lecture in my class with profanity just to get my goat. Perhaps it's Minnesota nice, perhaps it's my Christian identity, but cussing others out for their (often inadvertent) insensitivity is not my style.

How, then, do I have cancer? And how do I talk about it?

∽

"Your story is so inspiring."

Since the diagnosis, and particularly since narrating my journey with cancer in a public way on the CaringBridge website, I'm often told my story is an inspiring one.

On good days, I appreciate the comment. That friends and family are inspired by my story encourages me. On really good days, I even inspire myself.

I've also been surprised by those I've supposedly inspired. A former student who lost her husband to cancer told me my story gives her hope. A dear friend whose wife died of breast cancer regularly tells me I'm inspiring. The graciousness of those who've endured such tragedy is humbling. If our places were reversed, I wonder if I would be able to be inspired by stories like mine.

On bad days, however, I have difficulty seeing the word *inspiring* as applicable to my life.

One day in February I received an email from a scholar acquaintance of mine. He wrote that he had been following my story on CaringBridge and that he found my story inspiring.

That this message came in February doesn't bode well for a happy ending to the story. Graciousness wasn't mine that day, and after thanking him for writing, I told this well-meaning colleague that even though I might be an inspiration to him, I certainly wasn't an inspiration to myself. In fact, I found myself to be quite a downer.

Surprisingly, he never wrote back.

How do I have cancer? And how do I talk about it?

∽

"Isn't it amazing the lengths God will go to fix our gaze on him?"

Thankfully I have not been told very often that God gave me cancer. Maybe it's because I belong to a branch of American Protestantism that resists viewing God as the direct cause of all that happens in the world. Or maybe it's because it's intimidating to tell a religion professor how God is at work in her life. Whatever the reason, I'm grateful for the infrequency with which I have received comments that rest on assumptions I reject.

Still there have been a few.

Several months after the diagnosis I ran into a friend I had not seen in a while. After giving me a big hug, she stepped back and declared, "Isn't it amazing the lengths God will go to fix our gaze on him?"

This was a good day for me, but a bad day for an extended theological discussion about God's role in human suffering. I ran into the friend at a grocery store just as my daughters and I were heading for the car. *"Mmmmm Hmmmm!"* and a half-smile was all I could muster in response to her view of God as bringer-of-all-disaster.

What I wanted to say is that I seriously doubt God gave me cancer. That my friend, herself in the midst of a painful separation from her husband, would use the word *our,* however, gave me pause. She wasn't simply saying God gave me cancer; it seemed she believed that God had brought on the trials of her separation as well.

Even though I reject this view of God, I can imagine why my friend embraces it. We want there to be a reason for the pain, just as my students noted in our class on theodicy. It's true, too, that sometimes suffering is educational. The hard times *can* make us strong. A God whose judgment involves teaching us tough lessons about our sinful natures makes some sense.

But when it comes to undeserved suffering that threatens to destroy us—what people in my profession call *radical suffering*—this model of God as judge runs up against the image of God as loving and just. What if the cancer or the lymphoma that God supposedly ushers into our lives overtakes us? What if God's attempt "to fix our eyes on him" ends in early, painful death? Where's the love in that? Where's the justice in that?

I believe judgment—even wrath—is part of God's character. But to say that terminal diseases like cancer or AIDS are actually divine strategies to get us sinners to pay better attention to God means God's judgment outweighs God's love. That I cannot accept.

How, then, do I have cancer? And how do I talk about it?

∾

"God has his purposes for giving you cancer."

Closely related to "hardship as God's attention-getter" is the assertion that cancer is part of God's plan for my life. Cancer didn't just happen; God has reasons for bringing it into my life.

This comment came my way on a bad day. I shot back, "If that's the case, God sure as hell hasn't let me in on what that purpose might be."

It's quite possible that the friend who said this feels vindicated about the truth of his statement. I'm still alive; I'm writing about my experiences in ways that may be of help to others. I'll also admit to being a better person today than I was before the cancer. I'm more grateful, more appreciative of the gift of each and every day.

My friend could—and perhaps does—argue that all of these positive developments are proof of God's purpose for cancer in my life. I have cancer, I have been changed for the better, and now my story can be a blessing to others.

But here's where things get tricky. In spite of knowing I have inspired others and that I'm a more grateful person than I was before cancer, I would take it all back if I could. I would much rather be the person I was before cancer: a wife who believed she would grow old with her husband; a mother who planned to raise her daughters into adulthood; a daughter who assumed she would outlive her parents and in-laws; a sister, aunt, niece, and cousin who was just one of the family; a friend and neighbor who talked about something other than cancer.

Given the chance to turn back time, I would go back to being a little less grateful for my life, looking to embrace such gratitude more gradually. I would sacrifice the improved attitude to get back what cancer has stolen from me and from those I love.

That said, I can't discount the moments of grace I have been privileged to experience since cancer entered my life. I understand new depths of compassion, care, and love. I've glimpsed what living in light of unfathomable love must be like. I've been changed for the better, and as I don't have a choice but to be on this path, I'll take it.

I posted similar musings on CaringBridge, and was grateful for the courageous, honest response from a long-time friend from graduate school whose son has severe autism:

> As I read your words, I kept thinking about the journey we have gone through with our son. It is very different. Yet there are some deep similarities in accepting something so interlaced with both pain and gift. I stand exactly where you do: it has offered us such a precious gift, been the door through which so much compassion and light has been offered and received, opened our whole family to seeing the entire world differently. Yet if I were in front of the mirror of Eresid [the mirror from Harry Potter that makes visible a person's deepest desire] I know exactly what I would wish for. But as you say, we're not given a choice. It is the way it is. So just like you, I'll take it.

To admit there's no choice in having cancer or severe autism is not the same as believing they were sent by God to serve some grand purpose. I doubt cancer has a purpose in my life, even as I attempt to make meaning in cancer's wake.

How, then, do I have cancer? And how do I talk about it?

❧

"Cancer is a gift."

I have heard people in remission call cancer a gift. I have heard them say they wouldn't go back to life before cancer, even if they could.

I haven't had any good days dealing with this comment. Knowing the odds are strong that cancer will kill me in the near future, I am unable to see—or embrace—the gift character of cancer. In fact, I am troubled that other cancer patients actually embrace this view. I asked my friend who lost his wife to cancer what he thought of the cancer-as-gift view. He smiled ruefully and said, "I bet none of those people have stage IV cancer."

Viewing cancer as a gift could be related to the seriousness of a person's particular diagnosis. Then again I have known women whose early stage cancer sent them spiraling into depression and into being consumed with thoughts of death. For some, cancer's a gift; but for many others, it's an ugly word with vicious consequences.

If I could see into the future and know I had thirty years of remission ahead of me, I imagine I would be more amenable to thinking about my cancer experience as life-changing in a good, gift-like way. If I could reasonably expect that cancer wasn't going to kill me before my daughters graduate from high school, I might be able to be grateful for the wake-up call. But right now? A gift? No way.

At the same time, life with cancer has been rich with gifts. Cancer just isn't one of them.

How, then, do I have cancer? And how do I talk about it?

❧

"You don't look sick."

Our family knew what it meant to have breast cancer long before I was diagnosed. My mother's journey with breast cancer took her—and to a much lesser extent, the rest of our family—deep into the land of oncology clinics, mastectomies, prosthetics, chemotherapy, and radiation. We knew the drill as well as anyone: you get breast cancer, you have surgery, chemo, and radiation.

This familiarity with the breast cancer drill was at the heart of my disorientation with my diagnosis. *I had a broken back, which was caused by . . . breast cancer? What? How was that possible?*

Since that fateful day, my family and I have been brought up to speed on stage IV cancer and what it accomplished in my body. The cancer started in the typical breast-cancer way: with a tumor in my breast. Due to the dense nature of my breast tissue, the tumor went undetected by mammograms not once, but twice. Doctors did not locate the tumor until after they knew from my back biopsy I had estrogen-positive cancer, until after the second mammogram failed to detect anything. They finally found the tumor with an ultrasound test, when they were determined to find what they already knew was there.

So I'm a woman with breast cancer. The problem is my path to diagnosis and treatment bears little resemblance to the breast cancer drill many of us know so well.

After detection, rather than start chemotherapy, my oncologist informed us that the most important task was to stop the cancer from destroying more of my spine. Toward that end, I underwent radiation on my spine while the tumor in my breast remained untouched.

Because the cancer had spread far beyond the breast, the breast tumor was a virtual non-issue in the first months after the diagnosis. This disinterest in the cancer in my breast was unnerving, particularly to those of us well acquainted with the breast cancer drill. The oncologist emphasized repeatedly that the focus of my treatment needed to be the cancer traveling my blood stream and lodged in my bones. The anti-estrogen drug Tamoxifen and the osteoporosis drug Aredia—then Zometa—were put to work to serve this end. Surgery and chemotherapy might be called to do their part, but not right away.

I'm a woman with stage IV breast cancer with a broken back as the defining physical feature of the illness.

Those who saw me in those early days after diagnosis could tell I was sick. I was constantly nauseous; I lost weight and had considerable trouble getting around. It looked serious; it *was* serious. I had stage IV cancer. There is no stage V.

But I didn't lose my hair or my breast, two telltale signs of a woman with breast cancer. And this messes with people's minds.

"You don't *look* sick," was a common refrain when others saw me for the first time since learning I had cancer.

On good days, I was pleased at this comment. After all, I don't *want* to look like I have cancer. My monthly treatments in the chemo room reminded me how bad life with cancer could be. That I look healthier than what one expects to see in a stage IV cancer patient came as welcome news.

The problem was I did have stage IV cancer, even if it didn't look like it. Even if I didn't look sick, I *was* sick.

On bad days, the *You don't look sick* comment stung. It seems that because I did not have the requisite indicators of breast cancer—a bald head, a missing breast—my situation wasn't as bad as they had thought. Sometimes I was tempted to respond, "You've no idea the hell I've been through. I'm more than qualified to be a cancer patient." Usually on bad days, when I was told I don't look sick, I insisted, "But I am. Very, very sick," and I would wait in silence for a response.

How, then, do I have cancer? And how do I talk about it?

∾

"I just love your CaringBridge site; it's soo great!"

My brother's creation of a CaringBridge site ushered my family, friends, and me into a new world of publicly narrated illnesses. My journal entries and the thousands of messages of support have become essential companions on my journey with cancer. I can't imagine a more effective tool for updating others on how I'm doing. The site has allowed me to tell my story in my own words to loved ones far and near.

Still, it's not an unproblematic tool.

I'm not a Facebook or Twitter user, but many people I know—and many who follow my CaringBridge site—are. Even those of us who are not plugged into those social networking sites still spend significant time online. This has been confirmed for me every time I post a journal update. Within minutes there are a dozen or more responses. If I post before going to work, I barely step foot on campus before running into co-workers who say, "We're so glad to hear the positive update!" or "Thanks for letting us know about the test results!" The immediacy of the connection via the CaringBridge site is unnerving and gratifying all at once.

A couple months after the diagnosis, a friend told me how much she loved my CaringBridge site. "It's sooo great," she cooed.

Had it been a good day I could have imagined what she meant: that CaringBridge is a wonderful way for me to keep her and others like her updated on my condition; that the expressions of love and care for us in the site's guestbook witness to an army of supporters; that the site is her link to the recent good news I was hearing from doctors.

But it wasn't a good day and I felt my cheeks flush. *I'd give anything NOT to have a CaringBridge site* was the only response that came to mind.

My friend's complement also spoke to my suspicion that some users of CaringBridge occasionally view it as another social networking opportunity rather than as a tool dedicated to updating family and friends of sick people. In raving about my Caring-Bridge site, my friend inadvertently supported my concern that the site sometimes gets confused with more innocuous networking tools for simply staying in touch.

At least for me, CaringBridge is not primarily a tool for keeping in touch; it's about letting family, friends, and others know how I'm doing with stage IV cancer.

How, then, do I have cancer? And how do I talk about it?

❦

"You need to post!"

As is the case with many users of sites like CaringBridge, I wrote often during the first months after the diagnosis. Then February arrived; I was in freefall, and my inspiring story became less inspiring by the day. Journal entries on the site became less frequent.

A week of no posts went by, and I started to hear about it. My husband, fielding the calls and checking-in of family, friends, and colleagues, was the first to say it out loud:

"You need to post; people *really* want to know how you're doing."

It wasn't a good day to hear this. *Too bad for them,* I told my husband.

If it *had* been a good day, I could have focused on how desires for a post from me was evidence of others' care and concern. Many people have told me that my explanations of the pain, struggles, and worries gave them guidance in how to pray for me. Others realized how they could help by reading my CaringBridge posts. The posts allow others to care for me.

But as time went on, I realized that public narration of my illness could at times be a burden as well as a blessing. Chronicling my journey has been cathartic for me; it has been helpful for others to read. But there have also been moments I have felt pressure to write when I was out of words.

As a perpetual student, I learned from these experiences. Gradually I became clearer in my posts about how I'm using the site. As my condition improved, I informed my readers I wouldn't be posting again for weeks or even months.

Some readers commended me for backing off from frequent updates, cheering me on as I attempt to regain some semblance of a regular life. Others expressed disappointment with my extended breaks between CaringBridge posts, telling me how my posts kept their thoughts and prayers coming steadily my way.

I would love for my ordeal with cancer to be over, but it's not, and my CaringBridge site readers know that, too. So I keep writing. Occasionally.

How do you have cancer? And how do you talk about it?

∽

"Just so you know, I don't 'do' CaringBridge."

While my CaringBridge site allows me to communicate with loved ones near and far, it has also attracted some readers I barely know. Some log on to CaringBridge because they know a family member or a friend who knows me. And I'm grateful for each person's support, regardless of how well I know them.

In stark contrast to persons I barely know reading my journal entries is the rarer phenomenon of people close to me *not* reading CaringBridge. Some friends and family don't read the site, and are less aware of what's happening in my life with cancer. Publically narrating my illness, I have found, can also nurture the illusory view that everyone I know has read my latest post. But I have discovered, in unsettling ways, that's not always the case.

One family friend finally visited for the first time about five months after my diagnosis, just as life was regaining a bit of normalcy. She stood in our entryway, car idling in the driveway, and told me she had been thinking of me.

I appreciated the visit, but battled the voice in my head that kept reminding me that this friend had not come to see me in *five whole months.* Just as I made the decision to be gracious and count the visit as a kind gesture, my friend pressed on, "And just so you know, I don't 'do' CaringBridge."

"I've had two other friends with cancer who both used CaringBridge, and after reading their stories last year, I've had my fill of CaringBridge journal entries. I just wanted you to know."

I gaped at her. *You drop out of my life when cancer comes my way, and now you stop by to tell me that you're not following my story?*

"CaringBridge allows us to update others on how I'm doing," I responded, struggling to keep my voice calm. "Because of the site, we don't have to spend our time telling the same story over and over again. It's also been an incredible source of support for us, knowing that others have been praying for and thinking about us."

My friend could tell I was upset. She told me again she was thinking of me and headed back out to the car.

How do I have cancer? And how do I talk about it?

❧

I ran into a university colleague in the one of the most popular congregating spots at our university for female faculty members: the women's restroom. This colleague and I don't know each other well, but she had signed my CaringBridge guestbook a few times, expressing her concern and encouragement.

"I want you to know," she said as we walked out of the restroom, "I read your CaringBridge site, but it feels a bit voyeuristic, like I'm eavesdropping on your life."

I looked at her, surprised at the response.

"But I'm concerned," she continued. "I want to know how you're doing, and I want to let you know you're in my thoughts."

I appreciated my colleague's honest admission of how we are all still working on what to do and what to say in the midst of a cancer diagnosis. She reminded me of what I always want to keep at the front of my mind: that none of us knows exactly how to have cancer; that none of us know just how to talk about cancer; and that we continue on in the midst of not knowing.

ten

The Trouble with Miracles

SPRING SETTLED IN TO Minnesota. I was finally sleeping. My back was growing stronger. Descending cancer markers testified to the Tamoxifen's efficacy in slowing the cancer in my blood. Soon I would undergo more tests to show us whether the osteoporosis drug was doing the same thing for my bones.

Still I had breast cancer, and it was hard to forget about the tumor in my breast.

My husband was especially anxious to get the tumor out of my body. He didn't come right out and say it, but it was clear he hoped I would get a mastectomy, maybe even have both breasts removed. He sought out opportunities to remind me that while his love for me includes my body, he would gladly trade my breasts for more time with the rest of me.

Other friends and family familiar with the breast cancer drill were anxious too. Some feared I was getting bad care; I had breast cancer; why weren't doctors dealing with the *breast* cancer? Some urged me to find another oncologist, one who would get the tumor out—now.

During our April oncology appointment, my husband and I peppered the oncologist with questions about the breast tumor— now that I had regained some measure of strength, wasn't it time to think about surgery?

The oncologist reminded us that it was soon time for The Big Tests—a breast MRI, a bone scan and CT scan. Before taking any more steps forward, she told us, we needed an update on what the cancer was doing in my body. After the tests, we could set up an appointment with the surgeon to talk about surgery.

Which meant I would likely need surgery over the summer. My husband smiled a relieved smile. He had predicted summer surgery during a recent conversation with me about summer vacation.

My passion for summer stems in part from love of our annual family vacation during the summer months. Before cancer, we had planned on a New England vacation for summer 2009. Our older daughter was born in Connecticut while I was in graduate school, but she hadn't been back since we moved away when she was five weeks old. We had promised she would get there by age thirteen, and with her thirteenth birthday just weeks away, I raised the topic of summer vacation with my husband.

After I made my pitch for the importance of heading to New England *this* summer, my husband shook his head. "I bet you'll need surgery this summer, and surgery is more important than any trip." I feared he was right; still, the thought of giving up the best part of summer made me ache with sadness; hadn't I given up enough?

The oncologist's nod to summer surgery seemed to seal the deal of no summer trip. But before I resigned from yet another life-giving event, I wanted my oncologist's opinion on the vacation idea. Did she think it irresponsible of us to travel out east when we had surgery to think about?

"You should definitely go on your trip," the oncologist responded, with her trademark nod of the head. "With the treatment you're on, it shouldn't matter whether you have surgery in June or July. Go on vacation and have surgery when you get home."

I grinned and clapped my hands while my husband pretended to smile, looking as if he had just heard a bad joke but that he needed to be polite about it. In my husband's eyes, the oncologist ranks a little lower than God, so he knew he had just been overridden: what she says, we do.

But this was no time for me to gloat on my vacation victory; we had more questions for the oncologist. Even though I knew the surgeon would have strong opinions about what kind of surgery was best for me (indeed, we had already been treated to some of his opinions), I wanted to know where the oncologist stood on my upcoming surgery. Did *she* think I should have a lumpectomy? A mastectomy? Bilateral mastectomy? I laid the smorgasbord of options before her, urging her to pick out which one she thought best for me.

"There are advantages and disadvantages to both lumpectomies and mastectomies," she responded even-handedly. And then, rather than narrowing the choices, she added another item to the buffet: "after The Big Tests, you might even decide to leave the tumor alone and not have any surgery at all."

For those of us who know the drill, leaving the breast tumor alone seemed not just inconceivable but irresponsible. A quick glance at my husband confirmed that while he and I disagreed over the vacation-first-surgery-second scenario, we were in agreement on the tumor: it needed to come out.

We did not make any headway with the oncologist on the type of surgery, but we did manage to reign in the side effects of the monthly osteoporosis treatment. Following the suggestion of my physician in-laws, I took ibuprofen and anti-nausea meds before treatment and continued taking them every four-to-six hours for two days after treatment. Just as with my radiation treatments, taking drugs before the treatment blunted the force of the effects. For the three days following treatment I felt mildly ill but was able to stay out of bed while the sun was up. This was a huge relief. If low-grade nausea was as bad as it got, maybe I could endure twenty more months of treatment.

As my back became less of a daily concern, I grew increasingly preoccupied with the likelihood of breast surgery. I felt overwhelmed with the choices: how would I decide about what kind of surgery to have?

I asked my mom her opinion. Having had a mastectomy almost twenty years ago, she was unequivocal: "I wish I had had both breasts removed," she told me. From the challenge of finding prostheses to match her remaining breast to the anxiety surrounding every subsequent mammogram, my mom regrets not being able to choose a bilateral mastectomy.

I could see my mom's point about the bilateral mastectomy. At the same time I had difficulty imagining myself making such a choice.

I was finally ready to do some research. I read books on breast cancer, lingering over the sections on lumpectomies and mastectomies. As I digested the stories and the statistics, I found myself haunted by the negatives of each procedure. A lumpectomy would get me seven more weeks of radiation. A single mastectomy would lead to the challenge of matching a fake breast to the real one. Bilateral mastectomies have become increasingly popular in recent years, but taking a healthy breast along with the cancerous is stilled deemed a "radical" choice. With a mastectomy, I would also have lymph nodes removed from my arm. Reading detailed accounts of post-mastectomy problems with swelling and possible infections led to more sleepless nights.

Still there was more. If I had a mastectomy, I would need to decide whether or not to have reconstructive surgery, to go with a prosthetic, or to go with nothing at all.

The more I read, the more disoriented I became. Yet I knew that tens of thousands of women have had lumpectomies and mastectomies and many of them are living full lives today. Why was this decision so paralyzing for me?

Around this time a woman from our church who herself had had a bilateral mastectomy invited me to coffee. When we met, she walked me through her own diagnosis of stage III breast cancer and the decision-making process that led to the mastectomy. She told me of her conversations with other breast cancer survivors, and how their stories impacted her decision to have a bilateral mastectomy without reconstruction. Five years out from the diagnosis, she was delighted to report being cancer free and told me she shared her story with me just as others had shared with her, hoping her journey with breast cancer could be instructive for me. She even offered to show me her breast-less chest, just as before her own surgery, another woman from our church had done the same for her.

This was my first experience with the sisterhood of breast cancer survivors. This woman's initiative in meeting with me—and even offering me a view of her chest—left me speechless. I stumbled through an expression of appreciation for her willingness to share so much with me.

Unfortunately, the more I learned the more unsure of my own path I became.

Why was this so hard?

Against my husband's better judgment, I decided to give the cancer counselor one more try. I wanted to talk through surgery options and hear her thoughts on why I seemed unable to achieve clarity on what kind of surgery I should have. I was frustrated with my apparent vanity: here I was, a stage IV cancer patient with a lousy prognosis for living and I didn't think I could bear to lose a breast or two?

"Losing a breast is a traumatic affair," the counselor observed. "You've been through a significant amount of trauma already. You need to consider how much trauma you can handle at one time. Remember: you can always decide later on to have a bilateral mastectomy, but once you have one you can't go back."

I felt lighter hearing those words. Reframing the choice in terms of the amount of trauma I could endure opened up new ways to consider what I was facing. Perhaps my resistance to a mastectomy did not stem from wanting to wear tank tops over the summer; rather it could be that I had met my trauma-quotient for the time being. Maybe I could start small—a lumpectomy—and keep my options open.

While we were still on the topic of breasts, the counselor asked whether I planned to get tested for the breast cancer gene. I told her that my oncologist seemed supportive of the idea but that it wasn't part of the immediate focus of halting the spread of the cancer. I relayed to her my own concerns about the test; knowing I had the gene had ramifications not just for me but also for my daughters, my mother, my brother and his family. I was dubious about what the genetic test would get me other than confirming my fears about what I may have passed on to my kids.

The counselor wasn't as insistent as the surgeon had been about getting tested, but she did tell me that knowing whether I had the gene could help me deal with the choice of what to do with the tumor in my breasts.

I left the cancer counselor ready to think more about the genetic test.

I did more research. I learned that recommendations for bilateral mastectomies increase with a positive test for the gene. More consultation with my sister- and brother-in-law and my walking friend who had, of course, researched the subject thoroughly, led to the following conclusion: I wanted to be tested for the gene and find out I didn't have it.

Of course it might not be that easy. But I was ready to take the first step toward testing: set up a meeting with a genetic counselor.

Prior to our meeting with the counselor, I had to complete an extensive family health history, not just about breast cancer, but also about health issues of many members of my extended family. My mother, aunt, and cousin, all of whom are breast cancer survivors, completed special forms detailing the type of breast cancer, the location and size of the tumor, and their current state of health.

The health history forms were accompanied by a letter that concluded with this warning: given the high cost of the test and the small percentage of people who carry the gene, patients who meet with the genetic counselor should be prepared for her to counsel against getting tested.

The day of my appointment, the genetic counselor was meeting patients in her office in the Gynecologic Oncology Clinic. As my husband and I waited apprehensively in the waiting room, a very pregnant, very bald woman emerged from one of the exam rooms. She cheerily bid farewell to the receptionist and smiled gingerly at our wide-eyed stares. After the door closed behind her, my husband and I exchanged solemn glances. *To go through chemotherapy for cancer while pregnant?* It never took more than a few minutes inside hospital walls before I was reminded that my new cancer-filled life could be even more dire than it was.

The genetic counselor was an effective combination of crisp, efficient, and empathetic. She had done this counseling thing for many years, and had developed graphs, charts, and visual aids to help her patients understand how genetics worked and what the test would reveal. It also was a relief to jump right in to talking about the test; she already had all my information so there was no need for me to tell the broken-back-to-stage IV-cancer story.

The counselor began with a review of my family history, showing us a map of my family members and pointing to the most relevant pieces in my cancer puzzle. Despite having several women in the family with breast cancer, she emphasized that lots of breast cancer in a family does not necessarily mean it's genetic, or at least the kind of gene that can now be identified.

We moved on to a pie chart of breast cancer patients indicating that at present, breast cancer seems to be inherited only about ten percent of the time with a mere five percent of the cases related to the BRCA I or BRCA II gene.

Putting all the information together, the counselor estimated there was about a twenty percent chance that I had one of the breast cancer genes. The question we turned to next was whether or not I should get tested.

The counselor brought out yet another chart, one that compared women with breast cancer who have the gene to women with breast cancer who don't. And this is where I heard for the first time a decisive reason for getting tested: that women with breast cancer and the BRCA gene have a greatly increased risk of ovarian cancer.

"And with ovarian cancer, we have no good way to detect it. By the time it's discovered, it's usually stage IV and beyond treatment." The counselor looked at each of us in turn. "If you test positive for the gene, I would strongly recommend removing your ovaries ASAP."

At this point my husband starting asking questions. Like me, he was leery of the test, in part because he feared the effects of knowing our daughters might have the gene, too. "Why not get the ovaries out as a precautionary measure without taking the test?" he asked. The counselor agreed such action was possible, but not desirable. "No need to take parts out unnecessarily," she cautioned.

The geneticist's response opened the door for my question about mastectomies.

"What's your opinion on whether or not I get a single or bilateral mastectomy?"

The genetic counselor responded without hesitation. "I would support your decision to have your breasts removed. I would also support your decision to keep them. With your stage IV diagnosis, you are—and will continue to be—monitored as close as is humanly possible. If more cancer starts to grow in your breasts, they'll find it early. You can always change your mind and get a mastectomy at a later time. But I don't see a huge hurry now."

As the interview drew to a close, the counselor concluded by saying that she would support and encourage me to get tested for the gene. Most likely I didn't have it, she reassured us, and getting a negative result would provide relief. If I did have it, the counselor counseled, I could take steps—like removing my ovaries—that might prolong my life. But she acknowledged that testing positive would bring with it other ramifications not only for me but also for my daughters and other family members. This could mean testing for them, as well as the psychological burden of knowing what having the gene could mean.

We thanked the counselor and headed home. By the time we drove into the driveway I had decided to be tested. Though my husband feared more bad news—and his ability to weather more negative results—he told me I had his support.

The following week I returned to the hospital for a simple blood test that would be used to determine whether I carried the breast cancer gene. Then all we had to do was wait.

∾

The third time I asked the spine surgeon about physical therapy, he agreed it was time.

My first visit to the PT clinic offered yet another occasion to recount how I broke my back. To my relief, I kept my composure as I moved from fracture to diagnosis to radiation to life without the brace. The therapist was young and energetic and took my news of stage IV cancer in stride.

After scribbling several notes on my chart, she escorted me to the workout area where we started with some basic exercises. All of them were painful, but it was a hopeful kind of pain; I sensed that if I kept at these exercises, I would gain a stronger back and with it, more normalcy in my life.

I also learned that success in physical therapy largely depends on the patient's commitment to doing the exercises at home, in between the PT sessions. I welcomed the homework assignments, hungry for anything that could strengthen my back. I did the exercises diligently, as often as permitted. Then I asked for more.

Progress came quickly. A couple weeks into the therapy sessions the therapist directed me to warm up on a stationary bike. I smiled as I climbed on the bike, recalling my almost-daily bike rides before the broken back. After five minutes on the bike, the timer sounded and the therapist motioned for me follow her to the exercise table.

My feet followed the therapist, but mentally I was still on the bike. I asked the therapist whether she thought I could start biking again. She shrugged, "I don't see why not."

I left the clinic and went straight to the bike in our garage. After pumping up the tires I climbed on and meandered down the hill toward the river road that winds along the Mississippi.

After what seemed like eternity with a back brace and forever in a Minnesota winter, here I was, riding my bike again. Reclaiming my life hadn't felt more empowering than in this return to the bike.

My back felt surprisingly good for the first few minutes of the ride. Then the pain gradually crept back into my lower back. By the time I admitted to myself that riding was painful I was a couple miles from home. I left the river road, heading in the general direction of home.

The pain increased. I gave myself a stern talking to. *Why didn't you stay closer to home on your first bike ride in eight months?*

On the way back home, I had to stop several times to stretch my back. At last I pedaled into our driveway. But the pulsing pain in my back wasn't able to deflate my soaring spirits. I had ridden my bike. All by myself.

Biking may have been about the only thing I was doing all by myself, though. For months, parents from my younger daughter's school had been bringing us meals and doing our laundry. When these same families started to deliver a second round of meals, I grew anxious. *This is too much*, I told anyone who would listen. I called one of the mothers responsible for organizing this brigade of help, thanking her profusely and letting her know that now that I was able to ride a bike, I was able to make dinner for my family again.

The mother I called also happened to be the leader of our daughter's Girl Scout troop and apparently she had just been reviewing the Girl Scout promise to be *considerate and caring* and *to help people at all times.* While she expressed delight over my ride to the river, she didn't buy my story that one bike outing qualified as reason to abandon the brigade.

"You don't want to push it," she said. "How about we move from three to two meals a week?" Before I could protest, the What Friends Do website calendar she had set up for me was updated and yet more school families were signed up to help.

Sustained by the food and care of so many, I continued gaining steadily in strength, stamina, and hope. I was thrilled at my progress. At the same time, as a university professor, my surge in energy came just at the time when my university colleagues were succumbing to the cumulative effects of an academic year of too little sleep, too much grading and too many meetings. It was as if my colleagues and I were passing each other on opposing escalators, mine going up and theirs going down.

But April's impending exhaustion did little to stop my coworkers from extending care to me. Friends from work offered support in unique and creative ways. One treated me to a walk at a conservatory up the road filled with the aroma and vibrant color of blooming spring flowers. Another—who likely had heard me talk one too many times about my passion for scrapbooking— sent me a book on scrapbooks and American culture. Yet another knit me a brightly colored scarf. The colleague who had asked Jesus for a favor for me filled my mailbox throughout the semester with chocolate from Israel, Scandinavia, and Switzerland.

Cards from close friends and from coworkers I barely knew found their way to my mailbox. Colleagues treated me to coffee and lunch. A former colleague who had moved to Chicago started sending me a steady supply of blueberries: dried, preserved, even covered in chocolate.

Just when I thought I could not bear to receive any more gifts, a friend stopped by before class and handed me an envelope. "It's spring, which means it's time for a manicure and pedicure!" I stared at her, my loss for words now a normal part of my day.

"It's a gift certificate to a salon. Have fun!" she sang as she headed off to class.

Students expressed their support, too. They stopped by my office, offering updates on their lives, telling me it was good to see me.

But especially when my advisees came to visit, they offered hugs along with stories of how my diagnosis had worried them. In quiet ways, they let me know how concerned they had been about me. One advisee told me about her prayers for me at the Western Wall during her study abroad trip to Jerusalem. The brief spurts of time I spent at school were punctuated by these daily gifts.

In addition to the visits I received emails throughout the semester from former students jolted by my diagnosis into expressing their gratitude for classes they had taken with me in the past.

I struggled to live as a recipient of such grace.

In mid-April, families from my daughter's school signed up for a third round of meals. I couldn't bear it. I called the Girl Scout leader and told her that she and the other families had done more than enough good for our family. Really, seriously, we could make our own meals again.

This time, my friend finally agreed to give the brigade a rest. With the end in sight, I submitted a note to the school newsletter, thanking the dozens of families who had brought us food and washed and dried and folded our clothes. We had long appreciated this school community, but the depth of care we received was beyond anything we could have imagined.

Just as a school family delivered the last meal, I made the mistake of telling my sister friend at the university that we were done with meals.

The next day another friend of mine from work knocked on my office door and handed me a piece of paper. "I hear you're out of meals. Your colleagues have been waiting for months to bring you food. Here's a list of who's bringing meals when between now and the end of the semester."

Recipient. Recipient. Recipient.

It didn't take long for me to realize that the meals from my colleagues allowed me to use my energy for other important events in May, of which there were many. My older daughter's History Day performance was headed to the statewide competition. State History Day fell on May 2, the day my daughter and my mother share a birthday. My parents decided to join us for the day and combine birthday celebrations with the drama of history competition.

Two of my daughter's close friends were also competing, so together our three families traveled in a pack most of the day. That my daughter did not make it to the final round did nothing to dampen our spirits. After the awards ceremony—where we learned that one of our daughter's friends was going to nationals—these friends and their families joined us for a festive birthday-celebration dinner at a local restaurant. We toasted the birthday girls, the state history day champion, and our fine state performers.

As our families laughed and ate together, I sat back, drinking in the scene: my daughter, thirteen years old that day, reveling in the fun with her friends; my mom, full of smiles on her birthday; all of us, together, savoring the moment. I could scarcely believe I was part of such a joy-filled day.

Two days later, with the celebratory birthday-history day weekend still fresh in my mind, I was back at the hospital, drinking dye and getting poked with needles in preparation for The Big Tests.

My sister friend spent the day of Big Tests with me. My husband had initially insisted he be the one to be with me, for he had been at my side for every appointment thus far and wanted to keep the streak going. But all the time away from his work was taking its toll, and when my friend offered to accompany me I encouraged my husband to take a pass, reassuring him that I had been through these tests before and that he would be with me later in the week when we would hear the results. He reluctantly agreed, entrusting me to the good care of my friend.

Minutes after checking in at the hospital, I was called back for an IV to start the injection of dyes. I warned the technician about my difficult veins. She looked at my arm. "They look good to me—this shouldn't be difficult."

Two failed attempts later—*You're veins are sooo rolly*—the technician requested help and the nurse was successful. I returned to my friend in the waiting room with red puffy eyes.

"What happened?" my friend asked, startled into high alert. I hesitantly told her they had trouble with my veins. "That's lousy," she said, settling down a bit.

I hadn't even had my first test and I was coming undone. It was going to be a long day.

Our next destination was the Imaging Center for the breast MRI. I had learned from the oncologist and the genetic counselor that as a breast cancer patient, I would have breast exams every six months—first a breast MRI, then a regular mammogram, then back to the breast MRI. Because the breast MRI is much more sensitive than the mammogram, breast cancer patients typically undergo the MRI exam once a year.

Knowing that mammograms had twice failed to detect my breast tumor, I asked why I couldn't have the breast MRI every six months rather than just once a year. The response was similar to why they don't use an ultrasound as a regular breast-monitoring device: too many false positives. The breast MRI, I was told, detects everything, and the lion's share of what it picks up is benign.

It didn't take long for me to be glad I would have this test only once a year. After I changed into a hospital gown, they directed me to lay face down in a crypt-like contraption with my IV arm uncomfortably sticking out to the side. They hooked my IV to a packet of dye and informed me I would be in the imaging crypt for forty-five minutes. I knew from past MRIs that I shouldn't open my eyes and I tried to think distracting thoughts during the long procedure.

Relieved to be brought out of the MRI machine I massaged my IVed hand as it throbbed with pain. My veins weren't cooperating on this day of Big Tests.

Thankfully the bone scan came next, a test where the technician is not interested in IVs. The patient lies on a padded board as the scan slowly makes its way down the length of the body.

After the bone scan, I visited my friend in the waiting room, letting her know I was almost done. Minutes later I was called in for the last test, the CT scan. I hurried after the technician. The technician hooked my IV up to the fluid. He started injecting saline solution, and my hand trembled with pain. The technician stopped the flow and examined my hand. "There's no way you're going to tolerate the dye if you can't even tolerate the saline. We need a new IV."

This news was enough to push me back over the edge. Through my tears I told him about my uncooperative veins. "I'll call in the IV team," he told me. "They'll get the IV working with your veins."

Learning there's such a thing as an IV team was the highlight of my day. When the IV expert arrived a few minutes later, he inspected the failed IV. As he prepped my other arm, he coached me, "After this, always ask for the IV team. Don't let others mess with you. We'll get it in and working on the first try."

True to his word, he got a new IV going on the first try. I became an instant IV team fan; I was tempted to create a team cheer. With a functional IV, we completed the CT scan quickly and I was ready to go home.

Realizing it had been a tough several hours, my friend feigned hunger and insisted we go out to lunch. Getting out of the hospital and on to other non-health related topics of conversation helped me move beyond the morning.

But it was a long wait from Monday to Thursday's oncology appointment when my husband and I would hear the results of

The Big Tests. Just when it felt as if time had slowed to half its normal pace, I received an email from the president of our college's student congress. She wrote to inform me that the student congress was presenting me with the Faculty of the Year award. Could I make it to their meeting the following day?

For a moment, the Big Tests and their impending results faded into the background. I wrote back to the student president, telling her I would be delighted to attend their meeting.

The student congress session began with acknowledgement of the faculty and staff awards. The student president introduced the staff member and myself. She read from the comments of those who nominated us, including my advisee, who had slipped her prayer for me into the cracks of the Western Wall.

In addition to the student congress meeting, my award was going to be announced at the university's Honors Day ceremony, a program where students, faculty, and staff are honored for their achievements. On this day of high ritual on our campus, classes are cancelled and faculty and administrators process in full regalia into the ornate church sanctuary across the street from the university. Parents drive in from across the Midwest; some students even dress up. It's a day to honor and to celebrate. Being Faculty of the Year in the eyes of our students gave me something extra to celebrate.

The Honors Day ceremony took place on Thursday morning, hours before I was to find out the test results. My husband and my parents made time to attend the ceremony so they could see me receive the award. My husband and I also needed to head directly from the ceremony to the hospital for my appointment. As the program moved through the student awards, I tried to keep my thoughts away from what news might be coming our way later that day.

The ceremony approached the last of the student awards and I could see my husband and my parents standing together at the back of the church. They seemed to prefer chatting with each other to listening to the awards for students they didn't know. As I studied them from my perch at the front of the church, I was surprised to spot my husband's parents enter the church and join the rest of my family huddled by the door. I had not known they were in town, much less that they would be attending the ceremony.

The student president stepped to the podium and announced the Faculty and Staff of the Year awards. As I rose to accept the award, some of my colleagues stood and applauded. A few students cheered. I smiled broadly, happy for the award and grateful to be standing before this university community that had held me up over the past months.

I returned to my seat for the announcement of the final honor, the Faculty of the Year award given by the college faculty to one of its own. Shrouded in secrecy, the awardee's name is revealed only at the end of the ceremony, after a detailed recitation of the faculty's accomplishments read by the vice president who carefully avoids pronouns or specific references to the faculty's discipline of study until the very end. As the references to accolades mount, faculty whisper guesses to one another in attempt to trump the surprise.

As I listened to the annual recitation of the mystery winner's accomplishments, the pieces began to fall into place. My husband and parents semi-hidden in the church alcove, my parents-in-law mysteriously showing up at the ceremony and now the list of activities that sounded increasingly familiar; after thirteen years of listening to impressive descriptions of colleagues' achievements, I was listening to a recitation of my own professional career.

When the vice president finally called my name, I returned to the podium, smiling in disbelief at the honor. This time, the entire faculty rose to their feet. I had not expected to be honored a second time—and honored I was.

I returned to my seat in time to process out of the church with my colleagues. Once outside I was greeted with an avalanche of hugs and handshakes of congratulations. My husband and our parents were quickly by my side, laughing and hugging me tightly, delighted they had done their part to keep the secret.

I would have loved to bask in the happy glow of the awards and my colleagues' and students' congratulations, but it was time—past time, actually—to head to the hospital. My husband and I ran to the car, me pulling off my academic robe as we went.

I arrived at the oncology reception desk ten minutes past my scheduled check in time, which earned me a stern look from the receptionist. I acknowledged her gaze solemnly, aware of my tardiness. After having my blood drawn, it didn't take long until we were called back to the oncologist's office. The technician took my blood pressure and temperature and told us the nurse would be in soon. A few minutes later, the nurse came in and took down information on my medication, level of back pain, etc. "Do you have questions for the oncologist today?" the nurse asked.

We told her we were anxious to find out the results of The Big Tests. The nurse jotted down a few notes. "She'll give you more specifics, but the tests all look good." She smiled and told us the oncologist would be in shortly.

My husband and I looked at each other and smiled hesitantly. "Good news is good," I said. But as neither of us really knew what looking good meant, we waited—albeit a bit less apprehensively—to hear more from the oncologist herself.

The oncologist entered, shaking each of our hands in turn as she does every visit. She took a seat and said brightly, "Let's get right to the test results. Everything looks really good overall. The hip, tailbone, and lower vertebrae all show signs of healing; there are two small spots higher up on the spine that look a bit suspicious, so we'll continue to monitor them." She looked at us and smiled. "The reports of the scans look really good."

The oncologist turned the page of the report. "The news from the breast MRI is perhaps the best news of all. We know from the ultrasound last December where your breast tumor was, but the MRI didn't pick up any tumor in that spot. It seems that the Tamoxifen has taken care of the tumor. It's gone. The MRI showed a very small lump on the right breast, which the radiologist is confident is benign. We can have it biopsied to make sure."

She looked up from the report, and concluded, "This is great news. You're doing really, really well."

"That's great." "Excellent news," my husband and I replied simultaneously. Beyond those responses, we both were at a loss for words.

The tumor, gone?

Once I could think straight, I asked, "If the tumor's gone, does that mean I don't need surgery in the summer?"

In typical doctor style, the oncologist began with a disclaimer, "Well, you could decide to have your breasts removed as precaution against more cancer entering through your breasts, but you don't need a lumpectomy, because there's no tumor to take out. And there's no rush toward a mastectomy since there's currently no tumor in your breast. So I'd say there's no need for surgery this summer."

In an instant, the decision I had anguished over was put on hold. I couldn't believe it. I exhaled longer than I had since the diagnosis.

We thanked the oncologist for her expert care of me over the past five months. After our meeting with her, and another round of the Zometa treatment, we headed back home to share the good news with our daughters and parents.

Our girls took the news in stride, likely unaware of its exceptionality. Our parents shouted with joy. After filling them in on the details of the test results, I sat down at the computer and updated my CaringBridge site. The journal began with:

> Thank you, thank you for all your many prayers, good thoughts, and acts of kindness that have gone out on my behalf this week! We just returned from the oncologist appointment, and it's mostly awesome news! First, the best part is that the tumor in the left breast that supposedly started this whole cancer business is gone. It's no longer there. The breast MRI couldn't find it. We're calling this the Tamoxifen-prayer effect. The tumor couldn't withstand the

power of both put together! This also means that I'm not in
need of any surgery in the immediate future—yay!

I summarized the rest of the test results, emphasizing the
positive results. I concluded the journal entry by returning to how
the day began with honors and how we now had even more to
celebrate.

I'm so very happy to be able to share this life-giving news
about my health with all of you who simply overwhelm me
(and my whole family) with your love and support. Thanks
so much, and thanks be to God.

My family and I continued to ride the wave of thanksgiving
and celebration throughout the rest of May.

The good news also gave us energy to relish in our daughters'
accomplishments. For instance, our younger daughter played the
lead role in a rollicking little musical called "Proud to be St. Paul,"
performed by the third and fourth graders at her school. On the
day she was cast as the lead, my daughter burst through the front
door, saying, "You'll never believe this: I got the main part!" Her
expression told me that in truth, *she* couldn't believe she had been
given the lead. It didn't take her long to move from apprehension
to anticipation as the day of the performance grew near.

I arrived at my daughter's school extra-early on the day of
the performance, saving the front six seats for our family. My husband and I, along with all of my daughter's grandparents, sat in
the front row to watch my daughter, all of us beaming with pride
and cheering exuberantly as my daughter rose to the occasion.
She had overcome significant adversity, and this time I couldn't
have been happier.

Days after the musical more good news arrived. After
returning to the hospital for a biopsy of the small mass the MRI
had detected in my right breast, I received the message the Breast
Center is happy to deliver: the biopsy was benign.

Not more than a few hours later, I received another happy call, this one from the genetic counselor. The genetic test had come back negative: no gene for me, no gene for my daughters.

After months of awful news, we'd hit a streak of great news, and we inhaled it gratefully. I described this fresh sense of gratitude on CaringBridge:

> Spring has been gorgeous in Minnesota, and I've been savoring my ability to bike, to be in the garden, to attend the concerts, ceremonies, plays, and end-of-the-year celebrations that fill this time of year. One writer who shared her journey of stage IV breast cancer described the heightened sensitivity she had to the beauty of life when she was close to death. There is something to that; this spring, sunsets have literally caused my heart to ache; being present at my daughters' spring events has overwhelmed me with joy; that life is a gift has never been more real to me.

This period of good news offered a much-needed hiatus from the trauma of the past five months. The reprieve gave me and my family time to reflect on how this diagnosis—and now the miracle of healing—had changed our lives, our faith, our perspectives.

My pastor father decided it was time to tell my story to his congregation. He told the story from his point of view, from the perspective of a devastated parent, of a person of faith who shouted out in anger to God. He also told of my slow and steady improvements and the inexplicable disappearance of the tumor in my breast. As the sermon moved toward its conclusion, my dad spoke these words:

> In thinking back on the past nine months, a story from Mark 2 keeps coming back to me. There was a small group of men who met together, four of them were able-bodied, and one of them was paralyzed. The four would get together to support the injured man, they would pray for him and hope that he could be healed. Thus far no results.

But one day they heard that this man named Jesus was going to be nearby, word was out that he had been healing people, and so the men developed a plan. They would put their friend on a cot, carry him to Jesus. When they would find Jesus, they would ask him to heal their friend. But when they arrived in the area where Jesus was teaching, there was a huge crowd around him. There was no way to even get close to him. It would have been easy for them to give up and go home, but friends like this never give up. They tried to think of a way they could bring their friend to Jesus.

Suddenly one of them had an idea: why not climb up on the roof of the house, cut a hole, and then lower the man to the feet of Jesus? What a great idea: raise the roof! You can just imagine the fuss this caused, noise, disruption, debris falling down, a serious protest by the owner of the house, and then this man being lowered by ropes to the ground.

The Bible says something fascinating at this point. It says that when Jesus saw the faith of the friends, when he saw the incredible faith of friends who would even cut a hole in the roof, it says he healed the man. When he saw the faith of the friends, Jesus responded. I have this same image in my mind and heart today, that the faith of so many friends brought Deanna to the feet of Jesus, it was the prayers for healing of so many that made a difference.

And for some reason, which we do not fully understand, Deanna experienced a miracle, the tumor disappeared. I know very personally and painfully this is not always the outcome, we have had family members and dear friends whom we have brought to the feet of Jesus and they have not been physically healed. We do not know why some people are healed and some are not healed. But when we pray for a miracle, and then we see a miracle, it seems that we should celebrate, we should give thanks and praise to God, we should shout our hosannas.

It is the role and responsibility of all of us to bring others to the feet of Jesus, especially those who are facing life-threatening situations. It is often when our faith surrounds our loved ones that people are actually healed. Or at least if they are not healed physically, they experience true spiritual healing, and they no longer see death as a defeat but rather as a victory. Who should you be bringing right now to the feet of Jesus, even if you have to cut a hole in the roof, so that he can see your faith and bring healing and new life to your loved one?

Our family is giving thanks every day for the doctors and nurses and other medical personnel, we are giving thanks to so many people who prayed for us and brought us to the feet of Jesus. We are celebrating that Deanna has such a resilient spirit, and we are praying that the rest of the cancer will also disappear.

The most powerful part of my dad's sermon for me was his acknowledgement of how I was carried to the feet of Jesus by my friends and my family. "Miracle" isn't too strong a word to describe what happened to me. Hundreds and hundreds of people have prayed for healing for me; profound healing has taken place. A miracle has occurred.

Shortly after my dad preached the sermon about my miraculous healing, the husband of a friend of mine died of stomach cancer. Diagnosed in November, just weeks before my own diagnosis, this fine, fit, fifty year old man was struck down with cancer and the ferocity with which it hit him didn't let up. Now, just months after the diagnosis, he was dead.

In the midst of my father's testimony of my disappearing tumor, he acknowledged that for reasons beyond our ability to grasp, many who are sick, many who suffer, do not survive. Friends and family bring loved ones to the feet of Jesus and they are not physically healed.

Of course I know this to be the case. As a theologian, I've wrestled with this reality for a long time.

But living it is different than thinking about it.

Faced with the news of the death of my friend's husband, the questions came:

Why a miracle for me and not for him?

Why did the Tamoxifen-prayer effect work for me and the surgery-cancer drug-prayer effect seem to fail him?

If anyone were to make the noxious argument that I had more friends and family bringing me to the feet of Jesus or that I was somehow more deserving of healing than he was, I would put an end to such delusional thinking by talking about his loving family, the army of supporters writing in to his CaringBridge site and the thousand-plus friends, family, and neighbors who showed up at his funeral.

As the early deaths of gifted, loving people make blisteringly clear, healing in the face of a terminal diagnosis isn't about just desserts. It isn't about God giving us just enough—but not too much—to handle. There's no satisfying explanation for why I'm still alive and my friend's husband is not.

In his sermon, my dad also suggested that perhaps those who are not healed physically experience spiritual healing. Perhaps they begin to view death as a victory rather than a defeat.

I do not pretend to know what my friend's husband was thinking in the days before he died. "I can't live like this," was what he wrote in one of his last posts on his CaringBridge site. Doctors told him he had reached a point where medicine could do little for him. A few mornings later, he didn't wake up.

Could it be that he had decided he'd had enough? Did he come to view death as a friend—if not a victory—rather than an enemy?

Perhaps. I don't know.

Why a miracle for me and not for him?

How can I celebrate my miracle in the wake of another's death?

There are no adequate answers to these questions.

In my struggle to move forward, I was taken back my professor-friend's post on my CaringBridge site just days after my diagnosis. While it's easy to talk about what's good, mediocre, even bad in our lives, he wrote, "the horrendous initially strikes us dumb. When we throw words at it, hoping to defend ourselves, the words fall flat."

I have yet to find words that don't fall flat when talking about the early, painful deaths of my friend's husband, and the deaths of so many others each of us could name.

But for my friend writing the post, flat words don't have the last word.

He concludes his message with this:

> It is the same at the other end of the spectrum. The sacred ties our tongues. Only true poetry can give voice to the emotions the sacred elicits. But no words, however deeply felt or carefully chosen, can do the topic justice. This much, however, is clear. The two ends of the spectrum are linked.

Cancer's destruction and my subsequent healing have given me access to the horrific and the sacred all at the same time.

And I try to be grateful to God for those who've mediated the sacred for me, even when it's in the midst of the horrific.

eleven

Moving Forward, Standing Still

IT WAS ALMOST SUMMER, which meant it was almost time for my sabbatical, a coveted gift of the academic profession.

Sabbatical time, a holy time for academics, typically occurs once every seven years. It's not a year off, but a reprieve from teaching and meetings and office hours that opens up space to research, write and rejuvenate.

Practically speaking, the timing of my sabbatical was coincidental; it had been seven years since my last one.

Theologically speaking, the timing seemed more providential than coincidental.

During my first sabbatical seven years before, my ideal life percentage was consistently above the ninety-five percent threshold. My husband and I even took to referring to the year as a time of *sabbatical bliss* for the entire family. Everyone benefitted from my sane schedule: our girls enjoyed a year off from after-school care; my husband's schedule wasn't interrupted by my many school-year evening commitments; we were even treated to a regular diet of home-cooked meals.

Perhaps this second sabbatical would be blissful too.

Perhaps it would offer us time to recover and to continue healing from the trauma wrought by cancer. With the miraculous vanishing of the tumor, there was much to celebrate.

And more days than not I was in a celebratory mood. A couple months earlier my husband and I were discussing my burial plot; these last days of May I was back to riding my bike and making family dinners.

Still as we looked ahead to the upcoming year, the word *blissful* sometimes seemed a bit strong.

Just as I was celebrating the disappearing tumor, the start to summer and the gift of sabbatical, my husband began to slip back down into the valley of the shadow. I watched helplessly as the tears returned to my husband's eyes, as he struggled to smile in response to positive remarks about my current condition.

During one of our regular evening walks through the neighborhood, he and I talked about our repeated transfer of emotional control: we rehearsed how he had fallen apart immediately after the diagnosis while I had remained strong; how he had regained his footing just as I had stumbled into the land of despair; and how recently I had passed him on my way out of the valley as he was headed back down.

Moving deeper into conversation as we walked, we both surmised that this trading places was likely the way things go when couples face traumatic events. One partner is immobilized by grief and the other keeps it together. When the immobilized one begins to get a grip, the other is granted permission to come undone.

It made perfect sense.

It was also exasperating.

How much longer did my husband and I have to be on this seesaw, where one being up meant the other was down? In this playground of emotions, I longed to abandon the seesaw and try the swings, where we could go up and down side-by-side.

But for the time being we were stuck in this wearisome imbalance and I knew there wasn't much to do other than wait until my husband had energy to push away from the ground.

Still I felt stronger every day, and summer, *summer,* was upon us.

For the past several years, our family's Memorial Day weekend had included a twenty-mile bike ride across the river and through the woods to a Minneapolis lake. We would start out in the morning and stop at a nearby waterfall before venturing over to our favorite Minneapolis lake for a picnic lunch. After wading in the still-cold lake water and watching new families of ducks swim leisurely by, we'd climb on our bikes and head back toward Saint Paul, stopping for an ice cream treat to fortify us for the last steep climb back to our house.

While I had resumed my daily bike riding, we were all aware that twenty miles was likely impossible for my back. I admitted as much, but resisted resigning completely from this rite of summer. My husband understood the importance of this ritual to me, so he told the girls, "We're going to do The Big Ride again this year, and we'll go as far as mom's back allows. Once she's had enough, we'll stop and have our picnic, then we'll turn around and head home."

The girls supported this plan. That we might not bike the entire twenty miles was not necessarily depressing news, especially for my ten-year-old.

On the morning of The Big Ride, we packed our lunches and pumped up our bike tires before heading out. The ride to the waterfall across the Mississippi runs downhill the entire way. No problems there.

After a brief hike across the bridge for a closer view of the falls, we returned to our bikes, merging onto the bike path that took us through parks and forests bursting with new-spring green, and alongside a quiet bubbling creek and past the shores of several small lakes. We rode at an unhurried pace, the rest of my family checking in with me at regular intervals to make sure my back was stable.

More than an hour of biking, my back was fairing better than expected. When we stopped for a water break, my husband studied me and said, "Ready to turn around?"

To everyone's surprise, I wanted to keep going. If my husband or daughters secretly wished I had been ready to turn around, they didn't show it.

Back on the bikes, we continued our journey to the lake. As we meandered by yet another lake, I realized we were only minutes from our destination. We had biked almost ten miles.

The picnic food tasted even better than usual. After the wading and observing of ducks, we retraced our route toward home. Dairy Queen was packed with customers enjoying one of the first warm Minnesota days. As we headed uphill for the home stretch, both girls pulled out in front, determined to meet the challenge posed by the final hill.

Once at the top, our younger daughter parked the bike in the driveway, and sprawled—exhausted—on the grass. My husband and I laughed together, delighted with what we'd just accomplished. Less than six months after the diagnosis, six months after it seemed my life would soon be over, here we were, returning home after a twenty-mile bike ride.

On this day, *bliss* didn't seem too strong a word.

∽

Not long after our bike ride the girls and I finished school and the four of us boarded a plane to Connecticut to begin our New England vacation. We flew into Hartford, hopped in a rental car and sped down Interstate 90 to New Haven.

Our first stop was the apartment building where my husband and I had lived our last two years in New Haven, the place where our older daughter spent her first five weeks of life. After years of anticipating this visit, our daughter was all smiles as my husband and I led her and her sister around the neighborhood, caught up in the memories of our New Haven life.

Later that afternoon, we visited the New Haven firm where my husband had worked a dozen years before. The evening was spent with old friends dining outside in the cool, fresh June air.

The next morning we drove north and east, into the mountains of New Hampshire and the rugged wilderness of Maine. We hiked, ate delicious food, swam, read, and delighted in our daughters' enjoyment of the quaint New England towns and the breathtaking scenery of the East Coast.

Sitting in the car as we returned to our hotel after a sterling day of mountain viewing and hiking, waves of gratitude washed over me—for my life, for my increasing health, for my family, for the beauty we had witnessed that day, for the gift of another vacation. After so much of the horrible, vacation offered so much of the beautiful. I glanced at my daughters in the back seat, and my husband seated next to me, and smiled through the tears.

Noticing my gaze, my husband placed his hand on mine, his grin betraying a deep contentment I hadn't seen for many months. The familiar rhythm of the family vacation was helping him to push up on his side of the seesaw.

The Memorial Day bike ride, along with our trip to the East Coast, ushered our family back into a level of normalcy we hadn't experienced since I'd broken my back. We returned from New England and fell into most of our regular summer routines—biking, summer camps for the girls, golf for my husband—with a few new additions as well: softball for my younger daughter and monthly oncology appointments and treatment for me.

Able to manage the side effects of the treatment, my monthly visits to the oncology clinic were much less traumatic than they had been at first. My cancer markers also continued to look good; so good, in fact, that the day after my July appointment, the oncologist called to tell me my marker number had dropped below the coveted number thirty-eight.

"You're now officially in remission," she said enthusiastically. "You're doing wonderfully."

Hearing the oncologist say the word *remission* was like a transfusion of relief to my body and spirit. The cancer was being contained. I could scarcely believe it.

For the first time since the diagnosis I let myself ima..
that I might be part of the twenty percent of those with stage IV
breast cancer who live beyond five years. Better yet, perhaps I'd
join a growing percentage of stage IV cancer patients who survive
more than five years. It was thrilling to think about. I thanked the
oncologist. I thanked God. Friends and family joined in as we
celebrated more good news.

As word of my remission spread, I'd get the occasional congratulations for beating cancer.

Even as I reveled in remission, the congratulations tripped
me up.

I didn't quite know what to say in response. Yes, the cancer
was currently inactive but the scans showed it was still camped
out in my bones.

There was no doubt that remission was where I wanted to be.
And it *might* be a significant step toward a cancer-free life.

Then again it might be a temporary rest stop on a journey
with terminal cancer.

Amidst the incredible news of remission, I began to feel
caught, caught in between the relief of having many awful months
with cancer behind me and a nagging fear that the worst was yet
to come.

Each morning I'd wake up grateful for my declining cancer
markers. I'd also wonder when the day would come when those
same markers rebound past the magic number thirty-eight.

I was delighted to run into friends and acquaintances and to
respond to their earnest, *How are you doing?* with a *Great, thanks!*
With each enthusiastic response, however, my mind involuntarily
flashed to a time when the response to such questions would be
far different.

I was thrilled that the Tamoxifen and Zometa treatments
had halted the spread of my cancer. But every day I'd worry that
the time was approaching when their effectiveness would wane.

My oncologist told us that only after these drugs have failed
will she resort to chemotherapy drugs; given my reaction to

radiation and to the osteoporosis drugs, however, she worries about my tolerance for the chemo.

I fear having to find out whether her worries are well founded.

When I confide in friends about my fears and anxieties, some ask whether I've considered attending a cancer support group. I tell them I've considered it but that I worry my challenges may differ significantly from those who've lost breasts or endured chemotherapy.

Our local newspaper featured a story recently on the only support group in the area for women with stage IV cancer. While most of the support group members are over fifty years of age, the article mentioned two younger members of the group, both of whom died early deaths from the disease. Whenever a member of the group dies, the article reported, the remaining members attend the funeral and sit together as a sign of solidarity, just as they had at the funerals of these two younger members.

I feared I wouldn't do well in that kind of a group.

Hearing I was in remission increased the odds of it being a blissful sabbatical year.

Then again, *bliss* may be too strong a word.

∾

I began traveling again for work, attending an annual meeting of religion professors in Montreal, Canada. I reveled in reunions with treasured friends and colleagues, many of whom had been in regular touch since the diagnosis.

One of the highlights of the conference weekend was dinner out with old friends in a lovely old-city restaurant. My friends toasted my health and treated me to two constants in our many years of friendship: delicious food and delightful conversation.

As our dinner group began a leisurely walk back to the conference hotel, one of my friends—who also happens to be a Catholic priest—and I broke off from the rest of the group to pass by the famed Notre-Dame Basilica a couple of blocks off our route. The cathedral was locked but the view of its illumined edifice was enchanting. My priest friend offered a running commentary on the cathedral as we walked around the perimeter. I'm captivated by church architecture and viewing Montreal's Notre-Dame with the help of my friend made the experience even more memorable.

On our way back to the hotel, my friend and I talked about my health. I reviewed the miraculous developments. I also acknowledged the daily challenge of keeping fear of the future at bay.

After a few moments of silent steps, my friend asked the night air,

"Do you pray for a cure?"

The question quickened my step. In the many months of talking cancer, no one had asked me this question.

"No," I said quietly after a long minute of silence. "It seems too audacious to pray for a cure."

After a brief pause, my friend's voice cut through the darkness,

"I think it's ok for you to pray for a cure."

Visited by my customary loss of words, I walked on, my eyes growing misty. To be granted permission by a priest—and a dear friend—to pray for a cure was like receiving a sacred blessing. I hoped some of my gratitude seeped through the silence.

That night I lay awake wondering why I'd never actually prayed for a cure.

Surely the surgeon's words to me just days after the diagnosis—*you'll never hear the word cure*—were partly to blame.

But there was more to it than that.

As a teacher and a theologian I spend much of my time thinking and talking about the gravity of human suffering. More acutely aware of depths of pain and sorrow than ever before, I realized that praying for a cure for my cancer when so many others suffer even more seemed too bold, too self-serving.

But my wise priest-friend granted me permission to pray—for a cure. Maybe I could muster up the courage to do as he said.

Not long after I returned home from Montreal, I received an envelope in the mail. A small medallion was wrapped in piece of stationary. *I stopped by the Notre Dame Basilica when it was open and lit a votive candle for you*, my priest friend wrote. *The enclosed medallion has been blessed for you too.*

My eyes moved from the note to the medallion. Etched on its face were the words, *With God all things are possible.*

After my trip to Montreal, I thought a lot about praying for a cure. I even managed to do it a few times.

But most of the time, the word *cure* eluded me.

My blessed medallion read, "With God all things are possible."

On good days, I believed that was true.

Other days I was afraid what I hope for isn't possible, that after a brief period of remission, my markers will rise and I'll need to get to work on letters for that black box.

Some days I shudder as I remember back to the bleakest days of life with cancer. Among the many things I hated about being sick, the most grievous to me was seeing my deteriorating condition reflected back at me in the people I love. Their sorrow fed my despair.

The prayers, love, and support of so many carried me through that time. My faith offered comfort. But what finally drew me out of the despair of those ugly days was the realization that my condition was beginning to improve.

While I work to keep myself focused on present experiences of bliss, I'm not always successful.

Fear of the future lurks in nearby shadows. In those shadowy landscapes I glimpse a time where remission had ended, where my health is shot. In this shadow future, I realize that this time, there will be no getting better.

If that shadowy future becomes reality, will anything other than despair be possible for me?

When I was sick, I hated being so out of control, so vulnerable, so weak.

In remission I'm terrified of becoming that vulnerable again; terrified to watch my dying through the eyes of those I love; terrified of being unable to find the words to say good-bye.

I try to trust that with God all things were possible.

But sometimes I get stuck. Stuck in between the gratitude, the grace.

And the grief.

twelve

The Grace of Many Feet, Many Hands

I KNEW I NEEDED to try and accept what my life has become rather than wishing for what used to be or worrying about what might be.

But acceptance of my fractured life isn't something I could do by myself. Just as with every step along this journey, I needed help. Lots of it.

Toward the end of my first remission summer, two life-changing gifts of grace came by way of many feet and many hands, and with them I began to imagine gradual acceptance of what is.

"I registered for the Breast Cancer 3-Day Walk this summer and I'd like to walk in your honor," my friend told me. He had done the walk years earlier, before his wife had died of the disease. Now, a year-and-a-half after her death, he was ready to walk again. This time he'd walk in her memory and in honor of a sister, another friend and me, all of whom had breast cancer.

Having walked the much shorter Race for the Cure events in honor of my mother, I could only imagine what kind of a gift my friend was offering me. I tried to express my gratitude.

The 3-Day walk, we learned quickly, required not only serious time and training but also substantial fundraising on the part of each participant. The Susan G. Komen Foundation hosts an online fundraising page for each 3-Day walker where they share their reasons for walking and where all donations are listed. On our friend's web page were moving tributes to his wife and the three of us in whose honor he was walking.

Through CaringBridge, I encouraged those following my story to support our friend's effort. As spring came into full bloom, friends, family members, and even a former student donated to his cause.

Soon it was August and time for the Breast Cancer 3-Day walk. We made plans to meet up with our friend the last morning of the walk. As the 3-Day weekend progressed, our friend called with updates at the end of each day, his narratives punctuated by reflections on life in the tent city where all the participants stayed during the walk. He talked of the long wait to get into the medical tent for treatment for blistered feet and of the poignant stories of commitment to walk in the face of mind-numbing adversity.

In preparation to meet our friend at mile forty-three of the sixty-mile walk, the girls and I planned to make a sign of support to cheer him on. I logged on to the 3-Day website for inspiration about what to write on the sign. As I searched the site, I came across the section entitled, *How to Support Your Walker*. I scrolled down the page, quickly realizing there were multiple avenues of support I hadn't even considered. We could have been there to send him off at the opening ceremony; we could have sent letters of encouragement directly to the tent city.

I was upset with myself for not having found this information earlier. We could have done much more for our friend if only we had known.

Thankfully there was still time to act. In addition to meeting him on the route in the morning, we decided to create a welcome home kit filled with lotion and slippers for the raw feet, movies and books to encourage sitting with feet propped up, and energy drinks to replenish the fluids lost during the sixty miles. My husband headed to the store for supplies while the girls and I got to work on the sign.

Our friend called early the next morning to let us know he had boarded the bus and expected to be at mile forty-three within the hour. The girls and I scrambled out of bed and into the car.

The pink mass of walkers came into view long before we found a place to park. Supporters lined the road, many of them waving signs, others ringing cowbells and blowing kazoos. As we approached the crowd, a volunteer handed us pink inflatable noisemakers so we could join in the cheers.

We found a spot close to the stream of walkers where we'd be sure to see our friend. The girls quickly mastered the noisemakers and began cheering the walkers as they passed while I held up our sign of support for our friend.

Even though I've participated in several Race for the Cure events, I was unprepared for the intensity of this event. The 3-Day is like the Race for the Cure on steroids. Everyone walking the 3-Day has raised thousands of dollars and most have spent months training for the twenty-miles-a-day pace. The women— and a few men—wore t-shirts paying tribute to loved ones taken by breast cancer. Several bald women walked past, leaving me to marvel at their courage—and stamina—to participate in this grueling event amidst treatment for the disease.

While many walkers were energized by the knowledge they were in the home stretch, others clearly struggled to keep walking. A few were in tears, emotionally and physically exhausted by the enormity of the event. One woman broke down when she caught sight of her family members lining the sidewalk. After a tearful conversation with what looked to be her father, the woman dropped to the curb as the man took out a pocketknife and cut a hole in her shoe, lessening the pressure on the growing blisters beneath.

I struggled to keep my composure as I took in the scene. Next to me my girls were energized by the power emanating from the hundreds of dedicated walkers. They whooped and cheered as each walker passed by, eliciting many smiles and comments like, "We're walking for girls like you!"

My daughters understood at a visceral level that these walkers were really walking for them, and they cheered all the louder. I tried to add my voice to their cheers, but for the millionth time words eluded me. Here I was, a stage IV breast cancer patient, standing incognito at the edge of the 3-Day walk to raise money for more funding for the disease I was fighting. I felt deeply indebted to these walkers. But I couldn't manage to participate in the emotional scene of support for people like me.

I was grateful to finally catch a glimpse of our friend. He waved energetically and stepped out of the line to give us all enthusiastic hugs. His face contained a mixture of excitement, relief, grief and satisfaction. He assured us that his blistered feet weren't that painful (which I doubted) and expressed his amazement once again over other walkers' willingness to share their stories with him as they walked.

After basking for a few moments in our words of appreciation, encouragement, and thanks, our friend returned to the sidewalk for the seventeen final miles. We waved goodbye and cheered him on as his feet joined the many feet of walkers decked in pink boas, glasses, and hats.

We had done what we had set out to do: meet our friend at mile forty-three. But the girls were in no hurry to go home. "I don't want to leave," my ten year old admitted. "Let's stay for awhile," my thirteen year old urged.

The endless stream of walkers was hypnotic. The girls continued to cheer as loudly as they could. But after an hour or so of standing, my back had had enough and the girls and I got in the car and returned home.

Later that afternoon, our friend called to tell us he had crossed the finish line. The elation in his voice was contagious. "Way to go!" we all yelled into the phone. We gave him time to get home with his girls and then my husband and I delivered our welcome home kit. It was a relief to see him back home, even as he needed his daughters' support to make it from the stairs down to the living room chair.

My husband and I tried to express to our friend how grateful we were to experience the 3-Day vicariously through his generous gift of participation on my behalf.

But still there was so much I couldn't say. As my husband and I left our friend's house, I realized that this friend had done much more than walked sixty miles or raised several thousands of dollars to help cure breast cancer.

What he had given me was much more than that. In his quiet refusal to let grief over his wife's death have the last word, he graced me with one of the most powerful visions of hope I've been given thus far. He carried the grief and the sorrow of his wife's loss throughout those many miles; at the same time, he moved forward, using his feet to be a blessing to me and to others.

On our way home, I couldn't yet locate the words to share with my husband what was starting to formulate in my head: that our friend's testament to life moving on was starting to temper my own fears about the future. Fears for my daughters' and husband's possible future without me were steadied by my friend's feet.

I'm not trying to discount the pain and grief that would visit my family if I were to die soon. But now I dare to hope that eventually they too would be able to put one foot in front of the other and walk on, just as my friend has done. Not in a forgetful way, but in a way that affirms the rich possibilities of the life they have yet to live.

Inspired by my friend's walk, I took a step closer to accepting my fractured-yet-graced life and what that life may mean for the future.

❧

Summer began to fade and our lives seemed to be less and less about cancer. Which was a relief. Most of the time.

Occasionally, though, the fact that I was in remission-limbo from cancer seemed to go missing from others' radar, which left me in limbo about how to respond.

Yes, I was doing exceedingly well. But the effects of the trauma of the previous months didn't give way easily.

Particularly challenging for me was the planning for my sister-in-law's upcoming fortieth birthday that seemingly ignored my still-healing back.

My sister-in-law had told us to save an end-of-summer date for a birthday celebration. In the meantime, my daughter's Girl Scout troop signed up to go camping that same weekend. Confident my sister-in-law's party would be an evening affair, I volunteered to chaperone the Girl Scout trip, eager to give back to this group of girls whose families had done so much for us over the past months.

As the camping-party weekend approached, my sister-in-law called to inform us that her birthday party would center around a noon-time softball game with family and friends.

This plan bore little resemblance to the birthday party my husband and I had envisioned. Not only did the softball game idea overlap with my Girl Scout chaperoning, but softball was also an activity in which I—given my back—couldn't participate. I told my sister-in-law that I'd still be frolicking in the woods with the Girl Scouts at the scheduled time of the game. But her response was uncharacteristically insistent: *This is my birthday party and I need you there.*

That night I complained to my husband about his sister's plans. "I made a commitment to Girl Scouts," I reasoned, "and besides, if I were to come to this softball party, I would have to sit on the bench and watch everyone else have fun."

My husband sat on the bed, massaging his forehead with his fingertips, a telltale sign he disagreed with what he was hearing.

"Listen," he began, "I realize this party is inconvenient, and that you won't be able to play in the game. But," he paused to look me in the eye, "this is not about you. This is about my sister and what she wants to do for her fortieth birthday."

The words lingered in my head after my husband grew silent and waited for a response.

As I processed what he had said, it dawned on me that behind my husband's words was the unspoken claim that the past nine months had been more or less all about me, and even though I had cancer—and even though I couldn't participate in a softball game—this party was not about me. My husband, who doesn't ask for much, was asking me to be gracious and let my sister-in-law have her day.

I debated protesting this injustice further, but after a few minutes of arguing with myself I reluctantly concluded my husband was right: this party wasn't about me. I should come home early from Girl Scouts to celebrate my sister-in-law's birthday. I wasn't happy about it, but I agreed with my husband that I should be there.

The anticipated weekend arrived, along with the last gasp of eighty-degree summer temperatures. After an action-packed evening and morning with a dozen ten-year-old Girl Scouts, my daughter—who had been asked by my sister-in-law to play softball too—and I piled in the car and headed back to the Twin Cities.

As we drove into the sunshine, my lingering resentment over the whole softball ordeal began to fade. The day's low humidity and cloudless sky were ideal weather for any outside activity; I had just spent a near-perfect morning with my daughter and her friends; and even though I couldn't play softball, I could smile from the bench at this last day of summer. It was my sister-in-law's birthday; this is what she wanted to do; and in the big picture, I was grateful to be around for it.

We met up with the rest of our family at my sister-in-law's. Bats and gloves packed in duffle bags stood ready to be schlepped to the nearby field. My family and I were informed we were meeting my sister-in-law's friends at the field. "They're always late," my brother-in-law informed us. "Hopefully by the time we've warmed up they'll show up."

The entire family meandered through the neighborhood on foot toward the local ball field. Just before we reached the field, my sister-in-law told us we had to stop and return a jersey to a neighbor. These neighbors happened to be friends of ours as well, so we agreed to say a quick hello before continuing on to the field.

Our friends opened their front door widely, broad smiles on their faces and nametags on their shirts. Worried we had interrupted some special gathering, my husband and I hung back, waving cautiously, ready to explain we were just stopping by to return a jersey before heading to the fields to play a birthday game of ball.

But our friends motioned us inside. "Welcome! So glad you could make it!" they cried out enthusiastically. My husband and I tried one more time to explain that we didn't mean to intrude and we weren't planning to stay. But my sister-in-law cut us off.

"This party they're hosting is *for you*," she said.

Not understanding at all what my sister-in-law had just said, my husband, my daughters, and I looked up the stairs into our friends' living room. It was packed with people, all of whom we knew. I did a quick mental check of possible reasons for such a party: it wasn't our anniversary; none of us had a birthday in the summer. Why would there be a party *for us* when we were supposed to be playing a birthday game of softball for my sister-in-law?

Our friends and family nudged us up the stairs. We were greeted by enthusiastic cheers of "Surprise!" along with smiles and laughter from family members, friends, neighbors, colleagues from work, and families from our daughters' schools. My older daughter, seeing her cousin standing next to my husband's coworker who was standing next to the mother of one of her friends exclaimed, "What a strange combination of people!"

It wasn't at all clear why this strange combination had assembled in our friends' living room. What *was* clear was that they had done so *for us*. And that was reason enough for me to start making my way around the expansive living room, hugging each person in turn.

Intent on greeting everyone in attendance, some of whom I hadn't seen since the diagnosis, I barely noticed the large quilt dominating the living room space.

As I finally made it around the room, our friend hosting this mystery party called for everyone's attention. Her remarks began with the claim that the idea for the party had come to her last February, during my bleakest days. Watching the cancer unravel our lives, our friend told us how she struggled to figure out what she and her family could do to help.

One morning, a vision of creating a quilt came to her. She considered this vision to be her marching orders and used the entries on my CaringBridge site to make contact with our friends and family members about making a quilt for us.

Our friend enlisted the help of a mutual interior-decorator friend to select a pattern and colors suitable for our bedroom. Then she recruited quilt-block sewers. Mailing the fabric, dropping off squares at various locations, even meeting prospective sewers clandestinely in coffee shops, our friend recruited a small army of sewers to help make her vision of a quilt for us a reality.

Over the summer, sewers sent completed squares back to our friend. A quilting frame went up in their living room. And utterly unbeknownst to us, my friend and her family hosted quilting nights throughout the summer, where friends and family gathered to stitch this quilt together.

Our friend concluded her remarks with a gesture to the quilt in the center of their living room. "Today everyone who worked on the quilt has come together to celebrate your healing and *to finish this quilt!*"

My loss for words was complete. I stared at my friend. I gazed around the room.

For the past eight months all these people had been working on a quilt for us?

How could we not have known?

So many people in the room had already done so much for us.

Could it be that they had really done this much more?

Struggling to overcome my shock, I managed some inadequate expression of thanks and moved to view the quilt. It was beautiful; full of bright, rich colors ready to complement our bedroom colors. In between the quilted flowers, sewers were stitching the hearts, crosses, and stars that completed the pattern.

After I had spent a few minutes at the quilt, marveling at the work and starting to hear the stories of elaborate secrets this quilt had demanded from everyone there, my sister friend from the university escorted me over to a table, pointing at the computer screen positioned on top. "Of course we had to scrapbook the story of the quilt," she explained excitedly. "The scrapbook is called 'Many Hands.' We asked everyone who sewed a square to send us a picture and we took pictures throughout the summer as the quilt came together. You'll get a copy of this digital scrapbook in a few weeks, once we add pictures from today and a photo of the finished quilt."

Again I was speechless. My husband and I watched the scrapbook slide show, stunned to see pictures of still more friends and family members sewing on the quilt.

How could we not have known?

What words could even begin to express our gratitude?

Over the next few hours, our family basked in the warm sunshine of our friends' backyard and in the deep love radiating from our dear friends and family who had all gathered to stitch together this masterpiece for us.

After the guests had left, my husband took my younger daughter back to Girl Scout camp while my older daughter and I relaxed on the couch with the host of the party. Our friend happily reviewed the many fabricated stories we had heard over the past months as people gathered to work on the quilt without our knowing. My friend even pulled out her laptop and showed us her file labeled *Quilt* that was filled with over a hundred email messages pertaining to the quilt and the party. Even more names of people who had worked on the project but couldn't make the party appeared.

The magnitude of this project took my breath away.

When I made another feeble attempt to express my gratitude for this unbelievable gift, my friend brushed it aside saying, "No, no, this is not about me. The quilt-making took on a life of its own. I've been blessed through the relationships I've developed along the way. This quilt has been a gift for us too."

I wanted to protest my friend's interpretation, having only an inkling of how much time, effort, and expense she had put into this project over the past eight months.

Pausing at the close of this most amazing day, I also sensed that my friend really meant what she said. The atmosphere at the party had been unlike any celebration I'd ever attended; the undercurrent of joy seemed to sweep everyone along with it. The quilt project, it was apparent, had become more than just a gift for us. The loving act of creating the quilt had given the sewers gifts in return.

As my daughter and I prepared to leave, my friend's thirteen-year-old daughter ventured her own interpretation of the day: "Maybe we can sleep in tomorrow instead of going to church," she proposed to her mom. "I think we had church today, right here, at the quilting bee."

I smiled at her insightful observation. I would let mother and daughter work out whether they would go to church the next morning, but our teenage friend was right: today's party had been a holy event.

My daughter and I made it back to my sister-in-law's house just as my husband returned from Girl Scout camp. There we learned even more about the detailed planning that got us to the quilt party. The softball game, it turned out, was pure invention intended to keep us off the scent.

"But what about your birthday party?" my husband asked his sister earnestly. I turned sheepishly toward my sister-in-law to listen to her response. After all, her day of celebration—a day that wasn't supposed to be about me—ended up being more about me than I ever could have imagined.

My sister-in-law smiled her characteristically good-natured smile. "That dinner next weekend you have on your calendar— that's the real birthday celebration."

My husband and I let out a collective sigh, relieved his sister would get her celebration.

My older daughter took the ride home offered by my husband, which left me driving the few miles home by myself through the dusky silence. At the quiet conclusion of this exquisite day, I savored the gifts of love, grace, and peace that the quilt and the party had given us.

Could life be any better than it had been today?

It didn't take long for me to answer this question with a definitive *No.*

And with my response came a realization: in addition to being the party of a lifetime, the quilting bee had also offered me a glimpse into what I am guessing the heavenly banquet must be like. No other image could do justice to its sacred, joyous quality.

And if that's the case—if what awaits us after this life is anything like the quilting bee—then getting sick again and dying no longer seem quite as foreboding as it had in recent days. An eternal summer at a quilting bee with those I love most. Why fear death if that's what's coming next?

As the sun dipped below the horizon, it dawned on me that the quilting bee had gifted me with even more than a glimpse of the heavenly feast. In addition to being offered reassurance about the future, I was simultaneously offered reassurance about the present.

What I mean is the quilt and the party also showed me was that I didn't have to die in order for the eschatological feast to begin. A taste of heaven was actually possible right here, right now.

What's more, it dawned on me that the opportunity for eschatological feasting hadn't occurred back in the days of my ninety-five percent ideal life, back when life seemed nearly perfect.

Instead the feasting came right in the middle of my fractured, grief-filled life.

And in this feasting amid the crying and the grieving, my life mapped the movement of the Christian gospel story in a way I never imagined it could: I have experienced firsthand a death and a resurrection. I have witnessed new life growing out of the ashes of death and destruction. It doesn't get more Christian than that.

Such conclusions on my part may lead some to think that I've changed my mind about seeing cancer as a gift. For the experiences of grace I've been privileged to have would not have happened had I not had cancer.

But my mind hasn't changed on the "cancer as gift" idea. Accepting this new life doesn't mean we need to be thankful for the suffering, the pain, the grief, the death. I still don't believe my cancer happened for a reason. It just happened. My life is still fractured.

And yet there's more. My friend's commitment to walk on in the face of death, the creation of a quilt by so many loved ones: these gifts of grace tilted the scales in my life from grief to gratitude.

I'm so fortunate.

I'm so blessed.

Even in the midst of a devastating cancer diagnosis and lousy prognosis, grace abounds.

thirteen

Hoping for More

As we sat on the couch reading the newspaper one fall morning after church, my older daughter set down the paper and looked at me with her quizzical gaze that accompanies the asking of big questions.

"When are you going to take your name off the prayer list at church?" she asked.

I was quite sure that my daughter's question was not hers alone. Other members of our church were likely asking the same thing. They had seen me during the dreadful days of February. Many knew of my remission. Folks from church likely looked at me now and saw someone who didn't look sick—at all.

In my daughter's question I heard a question I had even asked myself: "Why does the church still pray for me by name every Sunday?"

In response to my daughter's query, I tried out on her the answer I had formulated for myself: as long as I haven't heard the word "cure," my name stays on that list.

Being in remission is a wonderful thing, I told my daughter, but I'm a long way from being out of the cancer danger zone. I reminded her of the sobering eighty percent/twenty percent statistics of stage IV cancer (while my ten-year-old had never asked

143

about the details of the diagnosis, my thirteen-year-old had, and I had been honest with her).

"But I thought we were done with cancer," my daughter responded quickly.

My breath caught in my throat.

Hadn't she and I had the frank conversations about the grim realities of stage IV cancer?

How could she think we were done with it?

I looked searchingly for answers to these questions in my daughter's eyes. What I saw staring back at me was a look that told me that a healthy-looking mother was more compelling than any statistic she had been quoted back in the dark days of February.

"I hope to get to the day where I can ask for my name to be taken off the prayer list," I said as I stroked my daughter's arm.

But as of today, that's just a hope.

❧

This story began in fracture and ends in hope. But the path from fracture to hope is not a linear one; that my story ends with hope doesn't mean that the fracture has disappeared. I only need to run my fingers down the protruding path of my spine to realize that.

What ending in hope *does* mean is that I am learning to trust that grace is sufficient for today, for tomorrow and beyond. And that whatever happens, I know that grace will continue to accompany me on the rest of my journey through this life and even into the next.

On my sabbatical I wrote an essay called "Hoping for More" for a collection of essays about big theological topics like Christ, the church, sin, and grace. My task was to talk about eschatology, theologians' fancy term for God's promised future.

When I think about how cancer has changed the way I think and talk about hope, I have become aware of how contemporary theologians like myself have a lot to say about the present and seemingly little to say about the future—that is, about life after death.

I understand the reasons for the collective reticence. Christian history is replete with theologies that bypass earthly life for elaborate visions of life beyond. Many in my profession call for a Christianity that focuses more on today, especially on the injustices that mar our earthly existence. When talk of heaven results in devaluing life on earth, there's a problem. Christian faith is an expectant faith—but it's not simply an otherworldly one.

I get the desire to focus on the present. As a cancer patient who's also a theologian, I see a need for *more* theological work on how to talk cancer while talking faith. Indeed, the gospel's main attraction—Jesus—spends most of his time not just talking about God's future but in siding with the outcasts and healing the sick. We need to talk more about how contemporary incarnations of the body of Christ—like my experience with the virtual body of Christ made possible through the CaringBridge website—side with those with cancer and participate in the possibilities of healing in the here and now.

At the same time, there's more to the story.

And I wonder whether those of us who talk about God for a living do a disservice to the God of the Bible and to those who suffer when we limit our discussion to the present. After all, the Bible is full of promises of life with God not only in the here and now *but also* in life beyond the grave.

For all of us who struggle to trust in these promises—even in the midst of death-dealing conditions—hearing that there's more than just this terminal diagnosis or that life-shattering earthquake offers a word of hope. That the suffering of this world isn't the final word is an essential part of the gospel's good news.

The hope I'm talking about is a hope that begins with lament, in the cries of "Why Lord?" uttered in the midst of the sorrow and despair that fill our lives. Crying out to God is an acknowledgment of the sorrow even as it demonstrates we dare to hope for more.

But hope that arises from lament is often achingly ambiguous. We hope for the joy of a promised future with God even as we take stock of our current suffering, fears, and painful recognition of our mortality.

In the scientific postmodern age in which we live, people in my line of work spend significant time emphasizing the limits of knowing what lies beyond this life. While Christian faith talks of heavenly feasts and bodily resurrection, many of us wonder how to set these claims alongside the science of decomposing flesh or suspicions regarding the possibility of continued consciousness beyond death.

In light of these tensions that govern contemporary understandings of materiality and death, what should Christians be saying about our future life with God?

I don't have adequate answers to these questions either.

But even as I admit ignorance on the details, I nevertheless take heart in the fact that the biblical images of life with God are consistently and inescapably communal. The Apostle Paul asserts that in hope *we* have been saved; he also insists that nothing can separate *us* from the love of God in Christ Jesus. At the heart of the vision of life beyond this one is the affirmation of continued connection, of life in community.

My life-altering experiences of community since the diagnosis—from my graced relationships with my husband and daughters to my exponentially expanded notion of the church universal to the vision of the heavenly banquet in the form of a quilting bee—have convinced me that despite knowing little of the details about life with God beyond this one, I've been granted faith that it will look something like the banquets of grace to which I've already been treated.

∿

Fall gave way to the season of Advent. With the first year anniversary of my diagnosis on the horizon, the season was once again a time of darkness with smatterings of light.

⁓

The anniversary day finally arrived. To mark it I wrote this entry on the CaringBridge site:

> I write today on this 10th of December, remembering that a year ago today I was diagnosed with metastatic breast cancer. This has been an emotionally intense week—we've been revisited by the sadness and the grief this past year has brought, and aware of the anxiety and uncertainty that have become constant companions.
>
> But today is also a cause for celebration—indeed, a good friend has provided us with champagne to mark the passing of this day—and for gratitude for the healing, the remission, for the ability to enjoy a December free of hospital stays, and for all of you who have made this journey more bearable.
>
> The rest of my family left the house this morning wearing their breast cancer awareness t-shirts to mark this anniversary (it's below zero here; I'm wearing wool). In this Advent season, which is for us a time of hope, of waiting for God's gift of participation in and redemption of this world, we wear pink, thank God, drink some champagne, and set our sights on hope.

And as the months of remission persist, each one its own gift of grace, we know that the hope on which we set our sights is not fracture-free. Cancer shattered more than just two vertebrae. We continue to try and reassemble the pieces.

We hope and pray that our future includes many more years for me in this life.

But we realize that my future in this life may be brief.

We struggle to accept it all with grace: the gifts and the grief.